616.462 N251d 2013
Nash, Jen
Diabetes and wellbeing :
managing the psychological
and emotional challenges of
diabetes types 1 and 2

Diabetes and Wellbeing

WITHDRAWN

D0913429

WITHDRAWN

Diabetes and Wellbeing

Managing the Psychological and Emotional Challenges of Diabetes Types 1 and 2

Dr Jen Nash

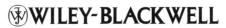

A John Wiley & Sons, Ltd., Publication

CUYAHOGA COMMUNITY COLLEGE
EASTERN CAMPUS LIBRARY

This edition first published 2013
© 2013 John Wiley & Sons, Ltd

Wiley-Blackwell is an imprint of John Wiley & Sons, formed by the merger of Wiley's global
Scientific, Technical and Medical business with Blackwell Publishing.

Registered Office
John Wiley & Sons Ltd, The Atrium, Southern Gate, Chichester, West Sussex, PO19 8SQ, UK

Editorial Offices
350 Main Street, Malden, MA 02148-5020, USA
9600 Garsington Road, Oxford, OX4 2DQ, UK
The Atrium, Southern Gate, Chichester, West Sussex, PO19 8SQ, UK

For details of our global editorial offices, for customer services, and for information about how to
apply for permission to reuse the copyright material in this book please see our website at
www.wiley.com/wiley-blackwell.

The right of Jen Nash to be identified as the author of this work has been asserted in accordance
with the UK Copyright, Designs and Patents Act 1988.

All rights reserved. No part of this publication may be reproduced, stored in a retrieval system, or
transmitted, in any form or by any means, electronic, mechanical, photocopying, recording or
otherwise, except as permitted by the UK Copyright, Designs and Patents Act 1988, without the
prior permission of the publisher.

Wiley also publishes its books in a variety of electronic formats. Some content that appears in
print may not be available in electronic books.

Designations used by companies to distinguish their products are often claimed as trademarks. All
brand names and product names used in this book are trade names, service marks, trademarks or
registered trademarks of their respective owners. The publisher is not associated with any product
or vendor mentioned in this book. This publication is designed to provide accurate and
authoritative information in regard to the subject matter covered. It is sold on the understanding
that the publisher is not engaged in rendering professional services. If professional advice or other
expert assistance is required, the services of a competent professional should be sought.

Library of Congress Cataloging-in-Publication Data

Nash, Jen.
  Diabetes and wellbeing : managing the psychological and emotional challenges of diabetes
types 1 and 2 / Jen Nash.
    pages cm
  Includes bibliographical references and index.
  ISBN 978-1-119-96718-7 (pbk.) – ISBN 978-1-118-48544-6 (epub) – ISBN 978-1-118-48543-9
(epdf) 1. Diabetes. 2. Diabetes – Psychological aspects. 3. Cognitive therapy. I. Title.
  RC660.N365 2013
  616.4'62 – dc23

                                                                                        2012042928

A catalogue record for this book is available from the British Library.

Cover image: © Lev Dolgatshjov / 123RF
Cover design by http://cyandesign.co.uk/

Set in 10.5/13pt Minion by Laserwords Private Limited, Chennai, India.
Printed in Malaysia by Ho Printing (M) Sdn Bhd

1 2013

CUYAHOGA COMMUNITY COLLEGE
EASTERN CAMPUS LIBRARY

Contents

Acknowledgements

Thank you to diabetes for teaching me all you have about myself. I've hated you, been angry with you and hurt myself because of you. But you've fostered in me a sense of resilience, courage and the tenacity to be myself. I wouldn't be the person I am today without you.

Thank you to the many, many people with diabetes I have had the honour of being connected with through my work at Positive Diabetes. Each one of you has touched my life, and your bravery in sharing your lives and experiences has enabled me to write this book.

I am grateful to my parents, Vera and Bill, who always instilled in me the value of education. This is the greatest gift you could have given me. Your values have changed the lives of the people who I have worked with; your lives have left a legacy.

Thank you to my dear sister Vanessa. You are a rock in my life. Your practical support and efforts made the writing of this book so much easier and smoother. But most of all, thank you for being a role model of faithfulness and unconditional love – and for loving me just the way I am.

Huge gratitude goes to my cherished friend Duncan, who always believed in me, encouraged me and spurred me on to write even when I doubted myself. Your unwavering faith in my potential made this book possible. Thank you.

Thank you to all the wonderful members of Marie-Claire Carlyle's Mastermind Group – you powerful women have been real role models to me and have encouraged me to step into a bigger vision of the impact I could have on the lives of people with diabetes. You inspire me.

Sincere thanks to all the team at Wiley-Blackwell for their dedication, believing in me and giving me the opportunity to write this much-needed book.

And finally. Thank you to everyone who has ever loved me, and who I have loved in return. You have taught me more than you know. I continue to be a work in progress – thank you for the gift of allowing me the space in your life to be that work in progress. It has been an honour to be a part of your journey.

1

Introduction

Life with diabetes can be hard work. Diabetes has been likened to a job – not just any job, but one in which you have to work 24 hours a day, 7 days a week, 365 days a year, with no holiday, no praise and no pay. I don't know about you, but I wouldn't stay working in a role like that for very long! But the individual with diabetes doesn't have the option of walking out or giving up; they have to keep 'working', day in and day out, for the rest of their life.

I really like this analogy of diabetes being like a job as I think it helps put into perspective how much of a struggle life with diabetes can be. None of us can do anything in life that requires effort over a sustained period without getting support and respite – and diabetes is exactly the same. You are probably reading this because you are someone with type 1 or type 2 diabetes yourself, a professional who works with individuals with diabetes, or perhaps a family member or loved one of someone with the condition. You are aware that although diabetes is a physical health problem, it affects the person in other ways too; and you want to know how to understand, help and support the person with diabetes. This book aims to offer both a person with diabetes and those around them a range of insights and practical strategies to help.

What is Diabetes?

Diabetes is a disease in which the body fails to produce or properly respond to insulin, a hormone that the body needs to convert food into the energy

Diabetes and Wellbeing: Managing the Psychological and Emotional Challenges of Diabetes Types 1 and 2,
First Edition. Dr Jen Nash.
© 2013 John Wiley & Sons, Ltd. Published 2013 by John Wiley & Sons, Ltd.

needed to live throughout daily life. There are two different types of diabetes – type 1 and type 2 – and each has its own causes, symptoms and treatments.

Type 1 Diabetes

The causes

Type 1 diabetes occurs when the pancreas stops producing insulin. There are a number of different causes of type 1 diabetes.

Problems with the immune system   Type 1 diabetes is an autoimmune disease. Your immune system is essential for fighting off infections. It works by attacking 'intruders' in the body that it doesn't recognize, such as germs. In diabetes the body reacts against and destroys the vital insulin-producing beta cells of the pancreas.

Abnormal characteristics on your chromosomes   There is evidence of certain abnormalities in the chromosomes, or DNA, of people with type 1 diabetes. Although these don't guarantee the development of diabetes, abnormal chromosomes are one factor to consider amongst others.

A virus   No one virus has been identified as responsible for causing type 1 diabetes; however, there is evidence that if a virus attacks the pancreas directly it can reduce its ability to produce insulin.

The symptoms

Increased frequency of urination   When the body isn't producing enough insulin, blood glucose levels rise, as the energy from food is not being converted into energy your body can use. The excess glucose ends up in the urine and makes it concentrated, then water is drawn out of the blood and into the bladder to reduce the concentration of glucose in the urine.

Increased thirst   Linked to increased urination. When you lose a lot of water in your urine, your body starts to dehydrate, causing thirst.

Weight loss   Glucose is being lost in the urine, so your body starts to break down muscle and fat in an attempt to obtain an alternative energy source.

Increased hunger The body doesn't have enough insulin to allow the glucose being consumed through food to enter the cells. Although the person is eating enough, the cells are malnourished, so hunger increases.

Weakness The glucose consumed from food isn't being used properly, which causes muscle cells to fail to get the energy they need from glucose. The result is physical weakness.

Treatment

Insulin Type 1 diabetes is treated by administering insulin, the hormone that is no longer being released by the pancreas. In the past, insulin was obtained from the pancreases of cows, pigs and some other animals. Now, however, almost all insulin is human insulin, produced in the laboratory. A number of different types of insulin are available, with short-acting and long-acting properties. So that the patient doesn't have to take many injections a day (four is the most common), different types of insulin have been developed to work for different periods of time.

Insulin can be delivered via a syringe, an insulin pen, a jet injection device or an external pump. Your healthcare team will advise you which option is most suitable for you.

Type 2 Diabetes

The causes

Type 2 diabetes develops when the body responds to insulin in abnormal ways. It usually occurs later in life than type 1 (although it is increasingly occurring at younger ages with rising obesity levels) and there are a few different causes.

Insulin resistance Unlike people with type 1 diabetes, those with type 2 do have some insulin in their bodies. People with type 2 are insulin-resistant: their bodies resist the healthy functioning of insulin. It is the combination of this insulin resistance with not enough insulin to overcome this resistance that causes type 2 diabetes.

Genetic causes Type 2 diabetes runs in families: a person with diabetes usually has a family member who also has the disease.

The symptoms

Fatigue   In order to feel energized, the cells in your body need fuel from the glucose provided by food. Fatigue occurs because the cells are not getting the fuel from glucose that they need.

Frequent urination and thirst   As the body can't make use of the glucose in the normal way, it needs to find another means of flushing it out of the system, so it stimulates thirst in order to ensure regular bladder emptying. The increased urination in turn leads to dehydration.

Blurred vision   The eyes are affected by rising and falling glucose levels: high blood sugar causes the lens of the eye to swell. Vision becomes blurred as the eye can't adapt quickly enough to these changes in the lens.

Slow healing of skin, gum and urinary infections   The white blood cells (responsible for healing infections) don't function well when there is a lot of glucose present in the body. This means the body is more susceptible to infections.

Genital itching   The glucose lost through the urine makes the genitals an ideal environment for yeast infections, such as thrush.

Numbness in the feet or legs   Type 2 diabetes affects the nervous system, and can lead to a condition called neuropathy, which causes loss of sensation or tingling and burning sensations in the feet and legs.

Obesity   People who are obese are more likely to develop diabetes, as the body has to work harder to convert glucose into energy.

Treatment

Diet   About four out of five people who are diagnosed with type 2 diabetes are overweight. Many people with type 2 diabetes can control their condition through diet alone. This means reducing calorie intake and eating a good balance of foods from each of the food groups: vegetables and fruits; protein, through meat, dairy and non-animal sources; carbohydrates, through bread, rice, pasta and cereal; and a small quantity of fats, oils and sweet foods.

Oral medication   There are a number of different oral medications for type 2 diabetes. Sulphonylureas are drugs that reduce blood glucose levels by making the pancreas produce more insulin. Metformin works by suppressing glucose production by the liver. Arcarbose blocks the action of an enzyme in the intestine, which leads to a slower rise of glucose in the bloodstream after meals. Glitazones are a group of drugs that directly reverse insulin resistance.

Insulin   Sometimes oral medication does not provide good enough control for the person with type 2 diabetes. In that case insulin may be required. Often one injection at bedtime is adequate, with more frequent ones added as needed.

What is the Emotional Impact of Diabetes?

Now you have a better understanding of the physical aspects of diabetes, we can move on to think about the various emotional and psychological issues that will be addressed in this book. There are a wide range of emotional factors that can impact the wellbeing of someone with diabetes – some of which affect people with type 1 or type 2 only, but many of which affect individuals with either type.

Dealing with diagnosis

The diagnosis of diabetes is a life event that has been likened to the experience of grief. In the same way as it is natural to grieve for a lost loved one, being given a diagnosis of diabetes can trigger a grieving for one's lost health. It is common to live life as if we are invincible, rarely considering our health or mortality. This dramatically changes when you are diagnosed with diabetes: you are suddenly acutely aware that your life is not without limits. You now have to rely on regular medication, frequent visits to a medical setting, and a team of doctors and nurses to keep yourself well. Chapter 3 will describe the stages of grief to help you better understand the process of managing diagnosis. By becoming aware of these different stages and recognizing the stage of the process that you or your patient or loved one may be in, you can manage the potential challenges better.

Depression and low mood

Psychological research has demonstrated that low mood and depression are very prevalent among people with diabetes; in fact studies have demonstrated that depression is approximately twice as common in people with diabetes as in people who are in good physical health. Life has its challenges and, for all of us, with or without diabetes, experiencing the whole range of high and low moods is part of the human condition. However, coping with a demanding condition like diabetes is an extra stressor to contend with, and it is very common to struggle with low mood at times. Chapter 4 will examine how to identify and manage depression and provide strategies to improve mood and wellbeing.

Guilt, shame and self-blame

Feelings of guilt, shame and self-blame can be experienced by people diagnosed with either type 1 or type 2 diabetes. For individuals with type 1 or 2 diabetes there can be the shame of being 'different' by virtue of having this health problem to contend with. For those with type 1, injecting and blood testing in public can be experienced as embarrassing and something that they would rather hide than engage in openly. People with type 2 diabetes may experience these emotions because they may have been aware that they needed to make changes to their health and lifestyle and they feel regret that they didn't act on this awareness in time to prevent diagnosis. Chapter 5 will discuss these emotions and how to overcome them.

Fear and anxiety

Fear and anxiety affect many people with diabetes. They can be divided into two categories: fear about factors in the here and now and fear of the future. Fear in the here and now may be anxiety over hypoglycaemia, fear of needles or simply the daily anxiety about the changes that diabetes causes in life. In terms of fear of the future, many people worry about the long-term complications and how they may have an impact in the years to come. Chapter 5 focuses on how to manage fear and anxiety in diabetes.

Using food to cope with emotions

For many people, both with and without diabetes, food can offer more than just fuel for the body. From birth, food is intimately linked to feeling safe and secure in the world, and in adulthood food can become a shortcut to dealing with difficult emotions. Many people go their whole lifetime using food in this way to a greater or lesser extent, and often without causing much harm. However, individuals with diabetes need to be more mindful of the role food plays in their lives, and that using food to cope with their emotions can cause problems. Chapter 6 will explain how and why these eating difficulties can develop and offer strategies to gain control of both food and emotions.

Communicating with health professionals

Developing a good working relationship with your healthcare team can go a long way towards making you feeling supported in your journey of managing diabetes. However, it's common for people to avoid going to their health appointments completely, or to feel a range of difficult emotions when they do go. Chapter 7 will explore the various ways you may be relating (or not) to your healthcare team and give you both practical strategies and emotional insights to help you see these relationships in a more helpful light.

Family relationships

Diabetes doesn't only affect the person with the condition – it has the potential to affect the whole family. Just as the person with diabetes can struggle emotionally, those around them can too. Family members can express their concern and worry in a multitude of different ways. Some loved ones may have a tendency to be over-involved with the management of diabetes, which can feel suffocating to the person with the condition. The opposite can also happen, when family members withdraw and seemingly ignore what is going on, leaving the person with diabetes feeling lonely and isolated. Chapter 7 describes these different ways diabetes can impact on the family system and offers strategies to help both the person with the condition and their loved ones.

Sexual difficulties

Difficulties with sexual response are a very common experience for people with diabetes and can affect men and women in differing ways. For the person with diabetes this can be a further setback: not only do they need to deal with all the other challenges of managing diabetes, now the part of their identity that could be expressed through their sexual relationship is hindered. It can feel like there isn't any part of life that isn't affected by diabetes. Chapter 7 will discuss the various ways sexual response can be affected by diabetes and describe both practical and emotional strategies to help.

How Does Psychology Help?

So we can see that there are a variety of challenges that can affect the emotional wellbeing of the person with diabetes. How can psychology help? Over the last century, a number of psychological theories have been developed that help us to understand our emotions and behaviours. The practical application of these theories through one-to-one counselling and therapy have been well researched and demonstrated to be helpful in offering insight and alleviating psychological distress. The theory that underpins the advice in this book is called cognitive behavioural therapy (CBT). In the NHS, CBT is offered as the treatment of choice for individuals who are struggling with both a chronic health problem (such as diabetes) and depression, and it has also been shown to be very helpful and effective for those who are experiencing emotional challenges more generally: anxiety, depression, anger, eating disorders and many others. CBT is built around the premise that thoughts are central to our emotional and behavioural responses. By examining our thinking styles and learning how to choose more helpful thoughts, we can choose more productive responses, which will improve our mood and wellbeing. Chapter 2 is devoted to teaching you everything you need to know about CBT in order to tackle the emotional challenges described in the remainder of this book.

Goal setting

Once you know the changes you want to make and have been equipped with the tools of CBT to help you implement them, you need goals to keep you on track. Goal setting is arguably the crucial ingredient of making any change in life, and failing to set realistic goals is one of the main reasons why life changes don't occur in the way we might want. Chapter 8 will outline how to set diabetes-related goals that work, and how to stay on track and motivated towards them.

Rewards

If you examine your life, there is probably very little, if anything, that you engage in for which there is not a 'reward' of some type. Diabetes is no different. Knowing that rewards are a fundamental of your diabetes care is often enlightening and encouraging; chapter 8 will describe how to use rewards as an integral part of your diabetes management.

Acceptance and mindfulness

Acceptance and mindfulness are psychological strategies that can be used in conjunction with CBT to good effect. Not only can they improve emotional wellbeing, they have also been demonstrated to improve diabetes control. Chapter 9 describes mindfulness in greater detail and includes practical strategies for implementing the mindfulness approach.

Staying solution-focused: managing setbacks

Setbacks are an inevitable part of the change process. In fact, expecting, managing and overcoming setbacks are arguably crucial elements to making any change in life. However, without this knowledge, setbacks can be the very part of the process that stalls people from making progress. Chapter 9 explains the importance of noticing and learning from setbacks to ensure they don't get you off track but, instead, provide an important part of the process that will enable you to make significant and lasting change.

How to Use this Book

This book has two broad aims. The first is to help you to better understand the ways diabetes can affect you emotionally, and the second is to equip you with new skills and strategies to manage your emotions in a different way. This greater insight coupled with the skills of CBT should, in turn, create more positive outcomes for your physical health.

I suggest you read the whole book through first, and then focus in depth on the particular chapters that are relevant to your situation. Although you may choose to ignore some of the chapters that aren't relevant to you, it is important to complete the exercises in Chapter 2 before doing any of the exercises in later chapters. This is because Chapter 2 teaches the skills of CBT that are fundamental to the material in the remainder of the book. Some of the exercises may look easy, but do complete them. When you actually try them they can be more complicated than they seemed at first glance. By trying them out, you are actively engaging with the material, which is crucial to make the changes that you want. Remember that many of the skills of CBT can be used in areas of your life not directly linked to diabetes, and many people report that the perspective it gives them allows them to enjoy their whole life more fully.

Further Reading

Gretchen Becker (2004). *The First Year: Type 2 Diabetes*. Constable and Robinson, London.

C. Fox, S. Judd and P. Sonksen (2003). *Diabetes at Your Fingertips*. Class Publishing, London.

C. Fox and A. Kilvert (2011). *Type 2 Diabetes at Your Fingertips*. Class Publishing, London.

R. Hillson (2001). *Diabetes: The Complete Guide: The Essential Introduction to Managing Diabetes*. Vermilion, London.

S. Jarvis and A. Rubin (2007). *Diabetes for Dummies*. Wiley-Blackwell, Chichester.

J. Rogers and R. Walker (2006). *Type 2 Diabetes: Your Questions Answered*. Dorling Kindersley, London.

J. Rogers and R. Walker (2010). *Diabetes: A Practical Guide to Managing Your Health*. Dorling Kindersley, London.

2

Cognitive Behavioural Therapy for Diabetes

The Importance of Managing Your Thinking Styles

Are you aware of the thoughts running through your mind right now? We have many thousands of thoughts every single day and it is likely that you rarely, if ever, pay much attention to them. However, research has demonstrated that our thoughts contribute much to our emotional wellbeing, and that if we can become aware of them, we can influence them, and therefore our moods and wellbeing.

Psychologists began paying attention to the role of thinking styles back in the 1960s, as a reaction to traditional Freudian psychoanalysis, which could often take many years to achieve long-lasting results. Aaron Beck (1997) was a psychiatrist who worked with patients with depression. He found that they experienced streams of negative thoughts that seemed to pop up spontaneously. He termed these 'automatic thoughts', and discovered that their content fell into three categories: negative ideas about themselves, about the world and about the future. Beck (1997) found that his clients would tend to accept these thoughts as true and valid, without reflecting on the authenticity of their content. He began helping patients identify and evaluate these thoughts and found that, by doing so, patients were able to think more realistically, which led them to feel better emotionally and behave more functionally.

CBT is now widely used to treat many emotional problems, including depression and anxiety, and is recommended as the treatment of choice

Diabetes and Wellbeing: Managing the Psychological and Emotional Challenges of Diabetes Types 1 and 2,
First Edition. Dr Jen Nash.
© 2013 John Wiley & Sons, Ltd. Published 2013 by John Wiley & Sons, Ltd.

for patients with both diabetes and depression. Even if you don't have depression, the techniques of CBT have been demonstrated to be extremely helpful in coping with the emotional experiences that often accompany the daily demands of managing a chronic health problem such as diabetes. Although many people work with a therapist, counsellor or psychologist to learn the skills of CBT, it is not essential. CBT can be used at home without a therapist, as long as the principles of treatment have been understood. CBT is a skill, and like any skill it takes time and effort to learn it well. It isn't a quick fix. By learning the skills and practising their implementation you will develop control over your moods, emotions and general wellbeing. This chapter will explain in detail what CBT is and the five-step process of putting it to use in your daily life.

What is Cognitive Behavioural Therapy?

According to the theory of CBT, any of our experiences has four aspects. There are the physical symptoms: what happens to us physically and the sensations we are aware of in our body. Secondly, there are our moods, emotions and feelings. Thirdly, our thoughts – what goes on in our mind: our thinking styles, images and memories. And finally our behaviours: the actions that we take or fail to take. These four categories of our inner experience all interrelate, so our thinking affects our body sensations, which affects our behaviour, which affects our moods.

So what does this mean in practice? Let's look at a case study. Eileen wants to lose weight and has been attempting to eat more healthily for a week. She steps on the scales at the end of the week to check her progress, and discovers that she has not lost any weight despite all her efforts. Eileen's thoughts may be, 'What's the point of trying? I have tried to eat healthily and I have not lost any weight! There is nothing I can do to change this.'

If Eileen is thinking these thoughts it is likely her mood will decline, and she may feel fed up, anxious or depressed. If she is thinking these thoughts and feeling these emotions, it is probable she will experience some changes in her bodily sensations, such as fatigue and irritability. If she is thinking these thoughts, feeling these emotions and experiencing these bodily symptoms, it is likely that her subsequent actions will be affected. For example, she may snap at a family member who asks how her healthy eating is going. Or she might decide to eat something sugary to cheer herself up.

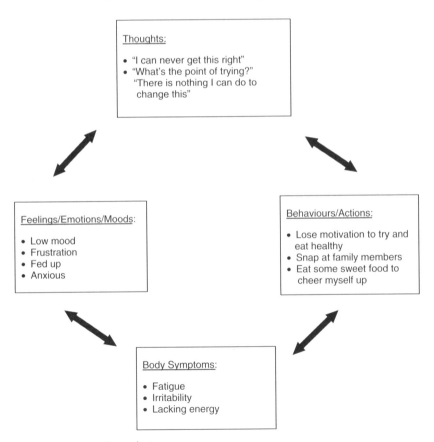

Figure 2.1　Eileen's CBT chart

According to the theory of CBT, all of these experiences – the thoughts, the emotions, the body sensations and the behaviours – interact to bring about a certain outcome. CBT focuses on our thoughts as playing the central role in our psychological wellbeing. Therefore by changing our thinking patterns we can change the emotions we are experiencing and the behaviours we are most likely to engage in.

So how can we change our thinking patterns? Perhaps you can identify with the example of Eileen and have had the experience of getting on the scales, realizing you haven't lost any weight and feeling disappointed. However, instead of reacting in a similar way to Eileen (Figure 2.1), you could think, 'Well, it's only been a week – I'll keep going for another week and see how I get on.' If you were thinking these thoughts it is likely you would have a different set of moods, a different set of body sensations, and therefore a different set of behaviours. Instead of snapping at your partner or deciding to eat a sweet treat to comfort yourself, you may think, 'This *is* frustrating, but what can I have for dinner tonight that is healthy and will help me stay on track to reach my goal next week?' You might ask your partner for a hug or to remind you of how good you'll feel once you've reached your goal.

This shift in thinking has the potential to affect profoundly both your emotional experience and your subsequent behaviour. This is key for good diabetes care, as much of the time you need to engage in certain behaviours (whether it be making healthy food choices, deciding to exercise or participating in your medication regime) to achieve the desired outcome. Focusing on your thoughts and replacing unhelpful thoughts with more supportive and empowering ones can help you to reach your diabetes goals and overcome the barriers that prevent you from behaving the way you would like in relation to your diabetes care.

How to Use CBT: The Five-Step Thought-Challenging Process

So how can you put CBT to use in your own life? There is a five-step process to using CBT; this section will guide you through it. Table 2.1 will help you.

Step 1: Ask yourself, 'What is the situation or event?'

When you notice your mood changing in relation to your diabetes, the first step is to increase your awareness about what exactly is happening. What is the situation or event? Many people believe that nothing has caused their shift in mood, and while this is sometimes the case (see Chapter 4 on managing depression, which discusses this in more detail), more often than not there *is* a trigger – either an internal or an external one. The skill is in increasing your awareness of the possible triggers that affect you. Examples of external triggers are stepping on the scales and seeing that you have not lost any weight this week. Or measuring your blood glucose and the result being higher than you were expecting. An example of an internal trigger may be thinking about your upcoming clinic appointment and feeling stressed because, last time, you felt you weren't really being 'heard'. Whatever the situation is, use Table 2.1 to write the situation down in the first row.

Table 2.1   Five steps to challenging your thoughts

Step	Question	Example	Your Experience
1	What is the situation or event?	Measuring your blood glucose level and it being higher than you expected	
2	What do you tell yourself? What are the thoughts you notice running through your mind?	What have I done wrong? I can't do this. I'm a failure	
3	What is happening in your body? What do you do?	Mood – hopeless Body sensations – dry mouth, thirsty Behaviours – snapped at my partner	
4	Challenge your thoughts: ask yourself some helpful questions	What is the evidence for and against this thought? Is thinking this way helping me? Are there other ways of thinking about this situation? If a friend told me they were thinking this way, how would I respond? Am I thinking in 'all or nothing' terms?	
5	Develop an alternative, balanced thought	'I have tried. Just because I haven't got the result I wanted it doesn't mean that I'm a failure' 'If a friend was feeling this way I'd help her see what she could do differently next time, or suggest she phones her diabetes nurse to ask for advice.'	

Step 2: What do you tell yourself? What are the thoughts you notice running through your mind?

Step 2 is to write down the thoughts that are running through your mind when you are in this situation. At first it is likely that you will draw a blank when trying to think about your thoughts. This is common. However, do persevere, as many people struggle in the beginning. You may worry about writing your thoughts down for fear of making them worse, or you may feel that they are unimportant or ridiculous. Again, these fears are normal. Remember that by identifying them you are taking the first step towards controlling them and your wellbeing. Typical thoughts are:

What have I done wrong?
I can't do this.
I'm a failure.
There's no point.
I never get it right.
I just want to give up.
I'm not coping.
I should be able to do this.
What's wrong with me?
I hate diabetes.
This isn't my fault.

Write the thoughts you have identified in the second row of Table 2.1.

Step 3: What is happening in your body and what do you do?

Step 3 is to think about what is happening in your body and the actions you take. In terms of body sensations you may be feeling irritability and fatigue, or you may notice your heart rate increase or your breathing become more shallow. In terms of moods you may feel frustration, depression, anger or hopelessness. In terms of behaviour you may lose motivation to eat healthily or test your blood glucose again for the rest of the day. You may snap at your partner if they ask you how things are going with your goal. Write these in the third row of Table 2.1.

Mood – hopelessness, frustration, depression, anger, fear, anxiety, worry
Body sensations – irritability, fatigue, heart racing, headache, increased sweating,
Behaviours – snapped at my partner, didn't test my blood glucose, ate more than I planned to

Putting words to your emotions can feel a bit alien when you first try, so here are some examples to help you:

Sad
Frightened
Happy
Anxious
Lonely
Bored
Jealous
Annoyed
Angry
Shy
Nervous
Embarrassed
Excited
Confused
Grumpy
Worried

Step 4: Challenge your thoughts

Step 4 involves beginning to evaluate your thoughts and starting to determine how much each one is serving you (or not). Challenge each thought by asking yourself some helpful questions:

What is the evidence for and against this thought?
Is thinking this way helping me?
Are there other ways of thinking about this situation?
If a friend told me they were thinking this way, how would I respond?
Am I thinking in 'all or nothing' terms?
Am I getting things out of proportion?
Is this a fact or an opinion?
Am I just dwelling on one bad aspect of this experience?

Write your answers to these questions in the fourth row of Table 2.1.

Step 5: Develop an alternative, balanced thought

The fifth step is to use the enquiries from Step 4 to decide whether the automatic thought is serving you and, if it isn't, to develop an alternative, more balanced thought. If you're not sure if it is serving you or not, I would like you to assume for now that it isn't! In the beginning, we usually have many more unhelpful thoughts than helpful ones. Examples of balanced thoughts might be:

'I have tried to get my blood glucose to my desired level. Just because I haven't got the result I wanted it does not mean that I'm a complete failure.'

'If a friend was feeling this way I would help her to think about what to do differently next time or encourage her to call her nurse to ask for advice.'

Write the alternative thoughts in the fifth row of Table 2.1.

This five-step process can be used to help you to identify and manage the thinking styles that may be impacting your emotions and moods in relation to your diabetes. If it feels difficult, don't give up too soon. CBT is a skill, and like any skill – such as driving a car, learning a new language or playing a musical instrument – you have to practise it in order to use it well. If you drive, it is likely that you remember how difficult and awkward it was at first. However, with trial and error and with perseverance you did learn what you needed to do, and in what order, and can probably now do it without even thinking about it. In the same way, by practising the skills of CBT on a daily basis you will become more tuned into your thoughts and be able to notice the presence of thoughts that aren't helping you. If you haven't already started, I want to encourage you to begin today. Turn to Table 2.1 and bring to mind an occasion recently when you felt particularly low about your diabetes. Work through the five steps.

The skill of thought challenging

The central aspect of this five-step process is the thought challenging in step 4, so let's spend a bit more time considering this. It is important to recognize that CBT isn't simply positive thinking. There is likely to be at least some truth to some of your usual ways of thinking about your diabetes, and we don't want to take a naïve approach of sticking our head in the sand and avoiding thinking about the negative sides to diabetes. The process of identifying and examining your thoughts in detail allows you the opportunity to evaluate how *realistic* they are. Often people who start using CBT report that their usual ways of thinking were overly negative and their new thoughts are actually more realistic, not necessarily particularly positive.

For example, someone filling in the table may realize that they are thinking, 'I must have perfect control over my diabetes.' But how possible is it to have perfect control, 100 per cent of the time, of *anything* in life? It isn't! A new, more supportive thought could be, 'I am doing my best to manage my diabetes well.' Another example of a typical thought could be, 'Any blood glucose result that is too high or too low means I have done something wrong.' The new thought could be, 'This blood glucose level can happen for a number of reasons, many of which may be out of my control.' You can see that these new thoughts are more *balanced* than the old thoughts.

There are certain categories of unhelpful thinking styles that everyone, with or without diabetes, has a tendency to engage in. Let's look at each of these categories of thinking (shown in Table 2.2) in turn.

Table 2.2 Thinking styles

Style of Thinking	Typical Thoughts
'Should' statements	Making a lot of rigid rules about diabetes, using words like 'should', 'must', 'got to' and 'ought to'
Making extreme statements	Using extreme words like 'always', 'never' and 'typical' to describe things
Bearing all responsibility	Taking total responsibility for things that may not be entirely your fault, such as developing complications
Putting a negative view on things	Tending to focus on the negative in situations rather than taking into account both the neutral and the positive
Catastrophic thinking	Predicting that things will go wrong, or that the worst will happen
All-or-nothing thinking	Evaluating in black and white instead of shades of grey
Over-generalizing	Because of one upsetting past experience, you conclude that this will occur again
Emotional reasoning	Taking a feeling as evidence of fact, such as concluding that you *are* a failure because you feel like one

'Should' statements   Many people with diabetes make rigid rules about their health behaviours using words like 'should', 'must', 'got to' and 'ought to'. Examples of this thinking style might be, 'I must have perfect diabetes control', 'I should be able to cope', 'I've got to get this right', I ought to be different'.

Extreme statements   This is using over-inclusive words such as 'always' and 'never' to describe things. For example, 'I never get it right' or 'I always get told off when I go to my diabetes appointments'. Is it true that you 'never' or 'always' have these experiences, or is it the case that sometimes you do and sometimes you don't?

Bearing all responsibility   This is a tendency to take total responsibility for things that may not be entirely your fault. Perhaps you blame yourself for making unhealthy food choices when there is limited choice available, for example at a party or a social event when you need to eat but there are no healthy food options. On these occasions you may blame yourself rather than accepting that you had to do the best you could in the situation you found yourself in.

Catastrophic thinking   Catastrophic thinking is the tendency to predict that things will go wrong or the worst will happen. For example, 'Nothing I can do will stop diabetes complications.' In reality we know that diabetes research has demonstrated that if we do our best to keep our blood glucose levels within the normal range, exercise regularly and eat healthily then we can actually do a lot to help minimize the effects of complications in the future.

Here are some examples of common thoughts that people with diabetes may have.

'I should take care of my diabetes perfectly'   Is this rule reasonable or possible? Does it set you up to fail? Can perfection even exist? An alternative, more balanced thought could be, 'I am doing my best to manage my diabetes well.'

'There is nothing that I can do to stop diabetes complications'   Many people who are frustrated with their diabetes will tell themselves this in order to opt out of having to even try. This is an understandable attempt to try to regain some control over a situation which can often feel quite uncontrollable. While it is true that no one with diabetes can predict if and indeed which complications may occur, by caring for your diabetes as well as you can today you'll be giving yourself the best possible opportunity for health in the future. An alternative, more balanced thought might be, 'I want to give myself the best possible health now and in the future.'

'High blood glucose results are a sign that I've done something wrong or bad' While this belief sometimes does have a basis in reality – like the times when you digress from what you know you should do in terms of diet, exercise and other health behaviours – this doesn't mean you are 'wrong' or 'bad'. Finding the stamina to keep caring for your diabetes 100 per cent of the time is extremely challenging. Often this belief is not only unbalanced, but also inaccurate. Some people go a long time criticizing themselves for a lack of 'good' blood glucose control, when trying out a different type or dose of insulin, changing meal times or exercising at different times may all be solutions to the problem.

Table 2.3 gives some further examples to help you.

Table 2.4 is a blank thought diary for you to complete with your own thoughts.

By now you will understand the basics of CBT and have started to apply it to your personal situation. The following chapters will focus on the specific challenges that affect people with diabetes, and address how CBT can help.

Table 2.3 Old thoughts, new thoughts

Old Thought	New Thought
I must have perfect control of my diabetes	I am doing my best to manage my diabetes well
Any blood glucose result that is too high or low means I have done something 'wrong' or 'bad'	Unexpected blood glucose results can happen for many reasons, many of which are completely out of my control
My diabetes comes first, my life comes second	My diabetes is a part of my life. I can achieve a balance with the support of my healthcare team
If I ignore diabetes, it can't hurt me	Diabetes is *more* likely to hurt me if I avoid thinking about it. Even spending a few minutes each day thinking and planning can be a great start
I hate the way diabetes controls my life	Investing some time and energy in caring for my diabetes will enable me to stay in control of my life and health

Table 2.4 New thoughts diary

Old Thought	New Thought

Reference

Beck, Aaron (1997). The past and future of cognitive therapy. *Journal of Psychotherapy Practice and Research* 6(4), 276–84.

Further Reading

David Burns (1999). *The Feeling Good Handbook*. Random House, New York.

R. Branch and R. Wilson (2010) *Cognitive Behavioural Therapy For Dummies*. John Wiley, Chichester.

W. Dryden (2011) *Be Your Own CBT Therapist*. Teach Yourself, London.

Dennis Greenberger and Christine Padesky (1995). *Mind Over Mood*. Guilford Press, New York.

3

Dealing with Diagnosis

Can you recall the moment you were diagnosed with diabetes? Perhaps it has been a very recent experience and is still fresh in your mind; or maybe it was a number of years or even many decades ago. Dealing with diagnosis is a process, not an event, so you may be surprised to learn that it can be as relevant for those who have had diabetes for many years as it is for the newly diagnosed. This chapter will outline how diagnosis can impact you, and how to better manage the process and overcome its potential effects.

Your Experience of Diagnosis

Regardless of the time that has elapsed since diagnosis, try to put yourself back to that moment now. Where were you? What was said to you? How was the news conveyed? What was the first thought that entered your head? Who was the first person you told? What were your feelings and reactions in the days and weeks that followed learning the news? You might like to make a note of your experiences below.

My experience of diagnosis:

_____

_____

_____

_____

_____

Diabetes and Wellbeing: Managing the Psychological and Emotional Challenges of Diabetes Types 1 and 2,
First Edition. Dr Jen Nash.
© 2013 John Wiley & Sons, Ltd. Published 2013 by John Wiley & Sons, Ltd.

Initial Shock Reaction

The diagnosis of diabetes can cause a state of shock. There is so much to take in: you have just found out you are suffering from a lifelong condition that does not have a cure. Your doctor probably told you a lot about medications and blood tests and diets and what to avoid, and your head was probably spinning as a result. You may have felt dazed and disorientated. It is likely you wanted to withdraw and felt anxious for the first few minutes after being told the news. All of these reactions are normal: most people feel this way to some extent.

Type 1 case study: Katie

Katie knew something was up. Her mother had had type 1 diabetes for as long as she could remember, and over the last few weeks Katie had noticed she was feeling more thirsty, needing the toilet constantly, and had no energy. She went to her doctor, who confirmed her fears. She had diabetes. 'Not now . . . not today . . . I'm not ready', she thought. She felt dazed, as if it was not really happening to her.

Type 2 case study: Jeevan

Jeevan had an infection in his toe which seemed to be getting worse, so he went to his GP, who did some routine blood tests. The next day, he was told he had type 2 diabetes. 'I thought there must have been a mistake! I don't know anyone with diabetes, and I'm not even that overweight!' Jeevan was angry and confused at how his life could be turned upside down overnight.

Whether expected or not, a diagnosis of diabetes is a shock. The experience of being diagnosed with diabetes is a significant life event. Many studies into the effects of diagnosis have likened them to those of grieving, and have demonstrated that the initial impact can cause grief responses and crisis reactions similar to a trauma (Edwards, 1987). In the same way as you may grieve for a lost loved one, the diagnosis of diabetes can trigger a grieving for your lost health. It is a very human trait to live life as if you are almost invincible, rarely considering your health or mortality. In fact, for emotional wellbeing, developing a certain amount of distance from thoughts of how fragile life can be is healthy. However, this can be dramatically challenged when you are diagnosed with diabetes. You are suddenly acutely aware that your life is not without limit. You now have to rely on regular medication, dietary and exercise routines, frequent visits to a medical setting and a team of healthcare professionals to keep you well. There can be a mourning process for the loss of the 'perfect self' who was unaffected by health problems (Kubler-Ross and Kessler, 2005).

Following diagnosis, it will take time to emotionally accept this new way of life. Accepting a chronic illness has similarities to accepting the death of a close friend or family member: it takes a lot of time and you may find yourself forgetting momentarily, and then experiencing a sinking feeling when the reality hits you. It feels like the 'non-diabetic' part of you has gone. You will need time to mourn your loss.

Below is an outline of the stages of grief, first described by Kubler-Ross (1997). Do you recognize any of the descriptions in your feelings towards diabetes?

Stage 1: denial – 'This can't be happening.'

Stage 2: anger – 'Why me?' 'It's not fair.' 'How can this happen to me?' 'Who is to blame?'

Stage 3: bargaining – 'I'd do anything to turn back time . . . ' 'If only I could have done things differently.' 'Just let me live long enough to see . . . .'

Stage 4: depression – 'I'm so sad.' 'What's the point?' 'I miss my old life.'

Stage 5: acceptance – 'It's going to be OK.' 'I can take control and manage this.'

Not everyone with diabetes will necessarily experience all of these emotional reactions, or in this particular order. However, it is likely that you can see the similarities between these thoughts about a diabetes diagnosis, and thoughts you may have had when faced with the loss of someone close to you. Just as the process of grief can be one that lasts for a long time, many people struggling with the diagnosis of diabetes oscillate between a number of these stages for many years, getting stuck at denial, or between anger, bargaining and depression, perhaps with small acceptances along the way.

Stage 1: denial

Denial functions as a buffer, or defence, after unexpected and shocking news. It allows you to collect yourself and, with time, mobilize other, less radical defences. You may find yourself daydreaming about a time before diabetes, about the news of a cure, about a coveted phone call that it was all a big mistake. Denial is defined as a refusal to believe something that is true, so according to this definition, you wouldn't be reading this page, or indeed anywhere near this book, if you were truly in the grip of diabetes denial, so well done for being one step ahead of some! However, denial affects lots of people with diabetes in subtle and not so subtle ways, and there are many levels and layers to denial. So how do you know if you are struggling with it?

Perhaps you identify with some of the following thoughts:

'Diabetes is no big deal; there are worse things I could have.'
'Why bother to care for myself? I'm going to die anyway.'
'My blood glucose level is out of control no matter what I do or don't do.'
'I just have a touch of diabetes', or 'I have borderline diabetes.'

You have permission to experience all of these thoughts about diabetes. Whatever your reaction to diabetes is a valid one. The problem with denial is that it is usually a defence against a place of pain inside. When you are physically wounded you need to both remove yourself from the source of pain (by pulling your hand away from the hot stove, for example) and spend time tending to the wound, Emotional sources of distress are just the same. You have to remove yourself from the place of pain – which denial allows you to do very effectively – and spend some time tending to the wound. Although tending to the physical wound can be painful, you know it is necessary to avoid further long-term damage. In the same way, bringing some of these painful feelings about diabetes to the surface may hurt in the short term, but it is important for long-term recovery and healing.

'Diabetes is no big deal; there are worse things I could have.' You are right, there *are* worse things you could be experiencing. There are a number of health conditions that cannot be treated and managed in the way that diabetes can. Thank goodness you haven't got one of these. However diabetes

is still a 'big deal', largely because the more committed you are to taking care of your diabetes, the better your overall health outcomes will tend to be.

'Why bother to care for myself? I'm going to die anyway.' Again, you are quite right, we will all die of something eventually. 'A short life and a merry one' can be the voice of denial talking, but it does not acknowledge the *quality* of one's life. We do not have a choice over when we leave this world, so it is not just the length of your life that is important, but the quality of the years you have remaining. By caring for your diabetes you will ensure that the years you have will be as healthy as they can be.

'My blood glucose level is out of control no matter what I do or don't do.' It can often feel this way, particularly in the early stages of managing the diagnosis. When you are still in the midst of getting used to how your food, activity, medication and lifestyle factors interact, you can feel pretty powerless, which is an upsetting feeling to have. It is easier to escape the upset by avoiding the facts. By evading gaining feedback about the actual level of your blood glucose, you sidestep the need to think about how you might begin to gain more control. This may also have a secondary (usually unvoiced) benefit, as changes you might need to make, such as making different food or exercise choices, are often uncomfortable to start engaging in. It is human nature to take the path of least resistance, so having this belief may help you to avoid having to make these changes.

'I just have a touch of diabetes.'/'I have borderline diabetes.' Thoughts like these are very common among people with type 2 diabetes who are not taking insulin, and can even be fostered by the reaction of the healthcare professionals involved at diagnosis. As Jarvis and Rubin (2007) point out, this is equivalent to telling a woman she has a 'touch of pregnancy'! The fact is that either you have diabetes or you do not, no matter what your current treatment regime. If feeling pleased that you do not have to inject is helpful to you, then good for you. The more you attend to your diabetes now, the less serious will be the consequences in the future.

Denial can actually have a positive role, particularly when you are first diagnosed or if you are going through a particularly stressful time in life. Being able to put diabetes in its own compartment for a time allows you to get on with life, and is a way of gaining back some control, until the particularly stressful time in life passes, or you are able to get used to the idea of being diagnosed with the condition. But whilst there can be some positive elements to denial, overall the negative aspects outweigh the possible benefits. Many studies have demonstrated that people who continue to use denial as a way of coping tend to have less good diabetes health than those who do not (Polonsky, 1999).

Stage 2: anger

Denial is replaced by feelings of anger, rage, envy and resentment. The obvious question is often, 'Why me?' You may find yourself looking at others in your life, perhaps even those you love dearly, and thinking, 'Why couldn't it have been them?' This stage can often be challenging for those around you as your anger is usually displaced onto everyone else: the doctor is no good, the dietician cannot help, the nurse does not understand, the reception staff are rude. Life is not turning out the way you planned; you now have diabetes, while everyone else is getting on with enjoying their (presumably healthy) life – the receptionist, the nurse, the doctor, the dietician. Even putting on the television can feel challenging: everyone, everywhere is having fun. Is no one noticing your pain? So you assert yourself and your control any way you can, by talking a little louder and letting your grievances show.

Anger gets a bad reputation in our modern society because of the damage it has the potential to cause, both to ourselves and to others around us. However, it is important to remember that anger is a natural human emotion that has evolved in us for a good reason: it has functional value for the survival of our species. Anger can mobilize our resources for corrective action when we have been wronged, denied or offended by another – when a boundary has been crossed. You have a right to feel angry at certain circumstances of your life that feel 'wrong', and diabetes is one of these. Life can feel challenging enough, without having a serious health condition like diabetes to deal with. Why should you be the one to have to struggle with coming to terms with this and all the difficulties it can bring?

Being aware of your anger is the first step to dissipating it. In what ways are you aware of your anger towards diabetes? Do you ever:

feel a surge of emotion in your stomach or heart area when you think about your diabetes?
feel more short-tempered than usual, with yourself or with others?
get more easily frustrated at life?
feel your heart racing or pounding, or get more sweaty in your palms and face?
feel a tendency to be a bit more bullying or blaming than usual?

physically destroy objects in your environment?

find yourself being more hurtful, by saying upsetting comments, or ignoring the feelings of others?

behave more selfishly, by ignoring others' needs or not responding to requests for help?

feel a sense of being 'speeded up', walking or speaking faster than usual, working too much, driving too fast or spending recklessly?

behave more unpredictably than usual?

How to tackle your anger

Write about your angry feelings. You could write a letter to your diabetes, expressing exactly what you think and feel. You can tear this up when you have finished, or even burn it (be careful to do this safely though).

Draw or paint your feelings. Even if you are not very artistic, just get some coloured pencils or pens and some paper and see what emerges when you start.

Imagine your diabetes as a person and sitting across from you in an empty chair. Tell diabetes exactly what you think of it.

Express your anger verbally. Shout, scream, swear if you feel like it.

Punch cushions.

Hit the bed with a tennis racquet or rolled-up newspaper.

Look for ways you can regain a small sense of control in your life and do these consciously. Even making everyday household decisions counts.

How to support a loved one who is angry If you are the loved one of someone with diabetes who is struggling with anger, do not take the anger personally. Try not to get defensive. It *will* pass. When the anger happens, try to take a deep breath, count to five in your head and ask your loved one what they need. If they are not sure make some suggestions: a hug, for you to express *your* anger at the diabetes in the ways described above, a walk in the park, some time alone. Look out for ways you can help your loved one regain a sense of control in life and offer these to them. Perhaps they could choose which music to listen to in the car today, what to do tonight or what to eat for dinner?

Stage 3: bargaining

'I'd do anything to turn back time . . . ' 'If only I could have done things differently'. 'Just let me live long enough to see . . . . '

Bargaining is the stage in which hope is invested in somehow postponing or delaying the reality of the diagnosis. There is a sense of regret inherent in this stage, and you are vulnerable at this time. You need to do much reworking of internal beliefs in order to come to terms with the trauma of what has happened. At this stage you may get lost in a maze of 'If only . . .' or 'What if . . .?' thoughts. Those with religious beliefs may pray, 'Please God, let me fall asleep and wake up realizing this was all a dream. I'll be a much better person, I promise.' You might have fantasies in which you are told that it was all a mistake, you do not have diabetes after all. Even if these daydreams and bargaining statements are not believed, momentarily they act as a reprieve from the pain of anger or depression. They can be an important attempt to restore order to the chaos you may feel your life is now in.

This is the stage when guilt is most likely to be felt. Getting diabetes is not your fault. As Becker (2004) puts it so eloquently, 'A lot of people may tell you that if only you'd eaten less sugar, or eaten less fat or exercised more, or eaten more fibre or smoked less, or done none of the things that 95 per cent of people do, you wouldn't have got diabetes.' There is further advice about overcoming guilt later on in this chapter.

Stage 4: depression

Being at the stage of depression may appear grave, and certainly it is natural to want not to feel depressed. But, however paradoxically, depression can actually be a sign of progress. It demonstrates you understand the certainty of the diagnosis, which is essential for resolution and progression. There can be a sense of hopelessness at this stage, and a tendency to disconnect from things and people that you usually enjoy and have affection for, including previously enjoyed pastimes and activities. Depression will be covered in much more detail in Chapter 4. If you feel you are really stuck at this stage, you might like to move ahead and focus on the material in that chapter.

It is a cliché, but a true one, that time is a healer. Like all times of mourning, this one will pass. Keep at the forefront of your mind that feeling down after any major change in life is completely normal. Nothing is 'wrong' with you; give yourself permission to be sad for a time.

How to support a loved one who is depressed   Distressing as it can be for those who are witness to it, this stage involves important emotional processing work. If you are caring for the person at this stage, do not be too quick to encourage your loved one to look at the sunny side of things or not to be sad. If they are allowed to express their sorrow, they will find final acceptance much easier.

Stage 5: acceptance

Acceptance is the final stage of the grief process; it signifies that you have come to terms with the diagnosis. Acceptance should not be mistaken for a happy stage. Rather, in acceptance, diabetes is allowed to be integrated with your identity. Although it will often remain unwelcome, it can become a part of you that can be cared for, rather than a stranger to be feared or fought. The strategies that follow in the following sections will help you to reach this state of acceptance.

Whether you are recently diagnosed or have had diabetes for many years, you may still be experiencing some of the different ways diagnosis can impact you. By becoming aware of the feelings you have towards your diagnosis and recognizing which stage of the process you are in, you can help yourself manage the potential difficulties better.

How to Manage the Emotional Impact of Diagnosis

Whatever feelings you have become aware of in connection to your diagnosis, you have a right to *all* of them. Every person's experience is unique and you have permission to feel every emotion you are experiencing: there are no 'wrong' or 'bad' reactions to the diagnosis. The first step to managing diagnosis is to learn to accept yourself as a person with diabetes. Just as you had value as a person before diabetes, you still have just the same level of value now that you do have diabetes. Accepting that diabetes is now a part of your identity is crucial, as is the process of learning to enjoy your life even if it includes the challenges of managing the demands of diabetes. Experiencing the emotions is important, and equally important is to know how to not let the overwhelming feelings paralyse you and keep you stuck in behaviours that aren't healthy for you. The steps to follow will help you with this.

Learning to LIKE yourself

LIKE is an acronym for the four steps to managing diagnosis better.

Learn   Educate yourself all you can about diabetes. Becoming familiar with the condition and its new vocabulary, and learning about all of the various aspects of managing the condition, allows you to integrate it as part of your identity and help you become an 'expert by experience'. No doubt you needed some element of training or teaching to be able to perform your occupation or learn a skill such as using a computer or driving a car.

You now call yourself a 'driver', 'computer-literate', or '[insert your job title]'. Diabetes is no different. You are likely to have been given some information about diabetes by your healthcare team: this is an ideal place to start learning the basics of the condition.

However, don't let your learning stop there. Borrow some books from your local library (join one if you need to!), and contact the diabetes charities (find further information in the Recommended Resources at the end of the chapter) to find out about local diabetes support groups and other useful resources these organizations offer. Obtain all the information you can from your healthcare team and ask them for recommendations of support or resources that other patients have found helpful. If you have internet access, you could join a diabetes internet forum run by one of the charities and learn from other 'experts by experience' who have been on a similar journey to yours and will be able to offer advice, hope and support, so crucial in these early stages of adapting to the condition. Start wherever feels manageable for you; you could set aside five minutes each day or thirty minutes at the weekend to do this.

Learning all you can about diabetes is not just for the newly diagnosed. When you have had diabetes for many years you may feel like you 'know it all', and in some ways you do: you are an expert in your own body and how diabetes affects you specifically. However, diabetes knowledge is advancing at an ever-increasing rate, so do not neglect to keep updated with all the new developments.

Inquire   Ask yourself what you can do to improve life with diabetes. At the top of a blank sheet of paper, write, 'My life with diabetes could be improved by .....' Your immediate response may be, 'Nothing!' or 'If I didn't have it!' That is OK; it is the resentment towards diabetes speaking, so there is no judgement of that being your initial response. Nevertheless, I want to encourage you to stick with this question for five minutes (set a timer on your watch or phone if that's helpful) and see what answers surface. Some things other people with diabetes have found helpful are:

Is there an educational course you can attend at your local NHS diabetes service? If you have type 1, then there are courses available to support you with your diabetes care. One of these, DAFNE (Dose Adjustment for Normal Eating), may be useful in teaching you how to alter your insulin requirements in line with your food intake. If you have type 2, a DESMOND course (Diabetes Education and Self-Management for Ongoing and Newly Diagnosed) can help you to gain greater insight into the management of your health. Chat to a member of your diabetes healthcare team about how to be referred to one of these free courses.

Would a dedicated kitbag for your diabetes equipment help you to feel more in control?

Or an attractive case with a design that reflects your personality?

A particular blood glucose meter that stores and memorizes your results?

An attractive notebook to record your blood glucose results?

A session with a dietician to explore different ways of managing your eating regime?

A system for remembering to take your medication or test your blood glucose (for example, putting a note on your bathroom mirror to remind you, or leaving your medication somewhere you will easily notice it, such as by the phone or next to your keys)?

Anything and everything that makes life with diabetes a bit easier is worth considering.

Get in touch with other people with diabetes, as they are the ones who will really know what you are going through. Although healthcare professionals know their stuff and are well-intentioned, they sometimes can't quite 'get it' (just as it is impossible to truly know what it is like to have lost a child, or be widowed, until you experience this yourself). Connect with others through a local support group, or, if you use the internet, an online support group.

Kindness Go easy on yourself and show yourself some kindness. It is common to experience a range of painful and powerful emotions towards your diabetes, as well as the anger and sadness that are inherent in the grief cycle. Guilt, rage, regret and numbness are all unnerving to contend with. These emotions can feel overwhelming. Try to keep reminding yourself that you have encountered an experience of loss and, as with any other loss, you cannot expect to feel your usual self straight away. Give yourself permission to feel the whole range of emotions. However, know that these painful feelings can and will pass. Formulate a 'kindness statement', keep it somewhere handy (in your diary or bag or by your bed) and read it at least three times a day. Ideas might be:

'I have a right to feel sad/angry/low/frustrated about diabetes but these feelings will pass.'

'I am going through a difficult life event, which will get easier to deal with over time.'

'I can choose to do something nice for myself.'

'Diabetes is demanding right now, but I have overcome other difficult challenges in life and diabetes will be the same.'

Express emotion   How can you express and let go of some of the emotion you are experiencing? Can you have a good cry? Talk to a trusted friend? Punch a pillow, do some exercise, write in a journal, see a therapist? You may be tempted to use alcohol, cigarettes or other substances to manage the overwhelming emotions that you may be experiencing following diagnosis. These substances are indeed shortcuts to feeling better in the short term, as they act on the mood centres in the brain to alter feeling states. It is therefore very likely that you will feel a greater desire to drink or smoke as an attempt to cope with these feelings and all of the practical challenges that accompany a diagnosis of diabetes. However, know that using these coping mechanisms for anything other than the very short term is not ideal. Again you can be kind to yourself and recognize that you are attempting to engage in a self-care strategy (this is often termed self-medicating, to reflect that it is a way of trying to heal emotional problems). Yes, they mask the root problem, but the root problem is still there to be faced. This is where techniques drawn from CBT can be helpful. (If you haven't already, read Chapter 2 to learn the basics of using CBT.)

Using CBT to Manage Diagnosis

Case study: Richard

Richard is 18 and has just been diagnosed with type 1 diabetes. He is about to start his first job after leaving school. Before the diagnosis he was excited about starting and was keen to save up so he could leave home. Now, though, he has been feeling upset and anxious about all the changes he needs to make to his life now he has diabetes. He is angry and feels life is unfair. None of his friends have to deal with this; why should he have to?

Case study: Parveen

Parveen is 41 and has recently found out she has type 2 diabetes, following a routine health check. As she has gradually put on weight over the years since her children were born, and both her parents had diabetes when they were alive, the news is not completely unexpected. She is sad though, and regrets not doing more to care for her health when she had the chance.

Step 1: What is the situation or event?

Richard   getting invited for a pizza and to the pub with my mates. Feel panicky about eating pizza and having some beers; not sure how it will affect my blood glucose.

Parveen   Out shopping for food, and aware of the need to make different food choices now. Sadness and guilt hit me, 'out of the blue'.

Step 2: What do you tell yourself? What are the thoughts you notice running through your mind?

Richard:

'I can't believe this is happening.'
'I'm angry that this has happened.'
'I hate my life now I have diabetes.'
'It's not fair.'
'I'm going to have to inject in front of them all.'

Parveen:

'If only things could be different.'
'What have I done to myself?'
'I'm so sad.'
'What's the point?'

Step 3: What is happening in your body and what do you do?
Richard:

Mood – anger, frustration
Body sensations – heart beating fast, shallow breathing, sweaty palms
Behaviours – bark at my mum when she asks me a simple question
    about what my plans are for tonight

Parveen:

Mood – hopeless, helpless
Body sensations – fatigue, feeling of dread in my stomach
Behaviours – want to leave the shop and cry, can't be bothered to carry
    on with the shopping

*Step 4: Challenge your thoughts by asking yourself some helpful
questions*

What is the evidence for and against this thought?
Is thinking this way helping me?
Are there other ways of thinking about this situation?
If a friend told me they were thinking this way, how would I respond?
Am I thinking in 'all or nothing' terms?
What other points of view are there?
How would someone else think about this?
How else could I think about it?
How would I think about this if I were feeling better?
What are the facts of the case?
How can I find out which way of thinking fits the facts best?
What is the evidence?
Could I be making a mistake in the way I am thinking?
Am I thinking straight?
Am I pressurizing myself?
Am I using the language of the extremist?
What is the worst thing that could happen?

Step 5: Come up with an alternative, balanced thought
Richard:

'I can't believe this is happening.' It feels difficult to believe that this is happening, but in the same way as I have coped with other bad news, I can and will cope with this.

'I'm angry that this has happened.' I've felt similar to this before (for example when I lost granddad, or got the news that I'd failed an exam), and although it felt very overwhelming at the time, I did get through it.

I have a right to feel angry that this has happened and I will choose to express this through [punching a pillow for 5 minutes, writing or drawing how I feel, talking about how I feel to my mum].

'I hate my life now I have diabetes.' Although I don't like diabetes, I like other parts of my life. I have a good group of friends and I'm about to start a new job. I am pleased that diabetes is not a death sentence and I can learn to control it.

'It's not fair.' It is not fair that I have diabetes, but I am glad it does not cause me physical pain, and it is not untreatable. I am grateful for that.

Parveen:

'If only things could be different.' Some days are easier than others. This is a difficult day. I'm going to do something nice for myself right now, like go to the park for a relaxing walk or sit and read a magazine with a cup of tea in the coffee shop.

'I'm so sad.' In the past, talking about my feelings sometimes helped me feel better. I could call my friend for a chat.

'What's the point?' Although I do not see it right now, there is a point to all of this. I will get through this, and maybe even grow stronger as a person as a result.

'What have I done to myself?' I don't like feeling guilty about the better decisions I could have made for my health. However, I can choose to make better choices now and in the future.

Formulating a kindness statement

Use the exploration you have just done to create a kindness statement to support you in the coming days and beyond. Remember that thoughts come very automatically and we are often not aware of their content from moment to moment. By formulating a kindness statement, you can actively choose what thoughts to think, and choose ones that will serve you.

'I give myself permission to feel [insert emotion you are feeling]. This is a normal and natural response to the diagnosis of diabetes. [Insert your alternative statement from Step 5 above.] In this moment I am going to choose to focus on [something good about your life, such as your relationship, your grandchildren, your friends, your job, your skills].

My kindness statement

_____

_____

_____

_____

_____

Dealing with Guilt, Shame and Self-Blame

A diagnosis of diabetes can often be accompanied by feelings of guilt and shame. You may have noticed some guilt response expressed in Parveen's thought 'What have I done to myself?' and shame in Richard's 'I'm going to have to inject in front of them all'. Guilt and shame are two closely connected emotions; this section of the chapter deals specifically with how to manage these.

What are guilt and shame?

Guilt occurs when you are in conflict about having done something you believe you should not have (or the opposite, not having done something you believe you should have). It is driven by a belief, accurate or not, that you have violated a moral standard. If you believe you 'should' have done something different or you 'ought' to have behaved differently, then you are likely to feel guilty. Shame too involves a sense that you have done something wrong, but it is more all-encompassing and cuts to the core of your self-esteem as a person. As Fossum and Mason (1986) eloquently explain, while guilt is a painful feeling of regret and responsibility for one's actions, shame is a painful feeling about oneself as a person. Like all of the emotions we experience, guilt and shame have evolved in us to aid our survival as a species. Our ancestors who felt guilty when they harmed another in the tribe reduced the chances of retaliation and thereby increased his survival prospects. In our modern-day lives, guilt and shame can be helpful emotions in certain contexts when amends can be made. However, in relation to coming to terms with a health condition like diabetes, they can be toxic, as there is little that is helpful or productive that can come from experiencing these emotions.

How do these emotions affect people with diabetes?

Feelings of shame and guilt are common for people newly diagnosed with diabetes. For individuals with both type 1 and 2, having a health condition can make you feel 'different' and there can be stigma attached to having a health problem. If you have type 1, injecting and blood testing in public can be experienced as embarrassing. If you have type 2, you may have been aware that you needed to make changes to your health and lifestyle and you feel guilty that you did not take action in time.

Overcoming guilt and shame

Managing and defeating problematic guilt and shame does not necessarily mean letting yourself off the hook if you have genuinely done something wrong. However, it does mean assessing and taking the appropriate amount of responsibility and coming to terms with whatever led you to feel this way. There are three steps: weighing personal responsibility (see Box 3.1), making reparations for any harm caused and self-forgiveness.

Box 3.1 Weighing personal responsibility: using a responsibility pie (Greenberger and Padesky, 1995)

1. Think of a negative event or situation related to your diabetes for which you feel guilt or shame.

   _____

2. List all the people and circumstances that could have contributed to the outcome. Place yourself at the bottom of the list.

   _____

   _____

   _____

   _____

   _____

3. Starting at the top of your list, divide the pie into slices, labelling them with the names of people or circumstances on your list. Assign bigger pieces to people or circumstances which you think have greater responsibility for the event or situation examined.

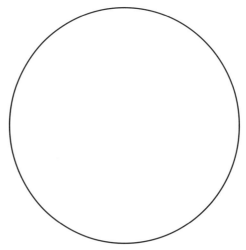

4. When you have finished, notice how much responsibility is yours alone and how much you share with others. Are you 100 per cent responsible? How does this responsibility pie affect your feelings of guilt and shame?

Parveen's responsibility pie

1. Negative event or situation leading to guilt or shame:
   Diagnosis of diabetes
2. People and circumstances which could have contributed to this outcome:
   Inherited genes – my mother and father had diabetes
   My early leg injury – means exercising is more difficult for me
   The death of my mum – we were very close and I got very depressed afterwards, turning to food for comfort
   Not always making healthy food choices
3. Parveen's responsibility pie (see Figure 3.1)
4. As you can see, Parveen decided that she *was* primarily responsible for her guilt about developing diabetes. Although her genes, damage caused by her early leg injury and her mother's death contributed, she felt she could have done more to be proactive about her health. She benefited from making reparations and self-forgiveness.

Making reparations

If you have hurt another person then it is important to make amends for your damaging actions. Asking forgiveness and discovering how you can

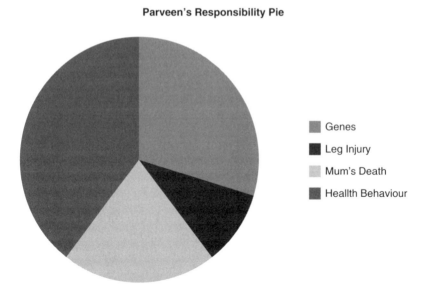

Figure 3.1   Parveen's responsibility pie

repair the hurt you have inflicted helps heal the damage caused. The same is true for guilt and shame that is directed towards yourself. Thinking about what you can do in the here and now to shift your feelings of guilt and shame can help you to heal.

Questions to evaluate guilt experiences (Greenberger and Padesky, 1995)

Can any damage that occurred be corrected? How long will this take?
Was there an even worse action or path I could have taken but avoided?

Parveen felt she could do her best each day to live a healthier life from now on. She was proud to recall that she has never smoked, even though when she tried it once she enjoyed it and her partner and many of her friends do. She also rarely drinks alcohol, which has helped her to stay healthier.

Questions to evaluate shame experiences (Greenberger and Padesky,1995)

Do other people consider this experience to be as serious as I do?
Do some people consider it less serious? Why?
How serious would I consider the experience if my best friend was responsible instead of me?
How important will this experience seem in one month? One year? Five years?
How serious would I consider the experience if someone did it to me?

Richard knew that if his best friend was diagnosed with diabetes he would want him to take care of his health and inject wherever he needed to. He knew that in a month this would be a lot easier, and he imagined that in five years he would barely be thinking about it, having done it so often. If he found himself being overly worried he could always go to the bathroom to inject until he got used to it.

Self-forgiveness

Being a 'good' person does not mean you will not make mistakes or will never do anything 'bad'. To err is human and perfection does not exist. Actions and behaviours may be less than perfect but that does not mean that you are a less worthwhile person. 'I made this mistake because I'm an awful person' could shift to 'I made this mistake during a really difficult time in my life when I didn't care how my actions would affect myself and others.'

Self-forgiveness involves recognizing your own imperfections and accepting yourself, including your shortcomings. It involves having a balanced view of yourself, acknowledging both your strengths and your weaknesses.

Practical Aspects of Dealing with Diagnosis

Telling others

Some people feel there is a stigma attached to having a health condition such as diabetes, and may want to hide the diagnosis from family, friends and colleagues. You will need to think about how to tell the other people in your life. There are individual differences in how you will want to approach this of course. Some people like to be very open and up-front straight away, and gain relief from those in their network knowing about this significant event. Others need time and space to come to terms with it themselves, so they can feel robust enough to respond to the inevitable questions that will come their way. You may find it difficult to tell others if you have always been the 'strong' one in the family, the one who coped during the hard times, and the one that took care of others rather than the other way around. Historically, men have been raised to be the strong one, and any sign of illness or emotional distress can be viewed as a weakness. This can cause you to want to keep your diagnosis private. Turn to Chapter 7 for ideas on communicating and expressing yourself more effectively, but in the meantime remember that many well-known public figures had or have diabetes and have not let the diagnosis hold them back:

Steve Redgrave, Olympic swimmer
Halle Berry, Oscar-winning actress
Winnie Mandela, Former head of the ANC Women's League in South Africa and Nelson Mandela's ex-wife
Elvis Presley, singer and performer
Mae West, actress
Elizabeth Taylor, actress
Douglas Cairns, first licensed pilot with type 1 diabetes to make a round-the-world flight
John Prescott, politician
John Peel, broadcaster
Jimmy Tarbuck, comedian

Ernest Hemingway, author
H. G. Wells, author
Sue Townsend, author

Informing your employer

There is no simple advice on this front. In an ideal world you would have an understanding and supportive employer who you would be able to tell about your condition. However, many people with diabetes feel a 'don't ask, don't tell' approach is a good one. If you are the breadwinner or the family are very reliant on your income then deciding whether to tell your employer can be a complex decision. Your boss might assume that diabetes means you will have to take a lot of days off work sick. Unfortunately, there can still be a lot of stigma associated with health conditions, and some ill-informed people have prejudices against anyone or anything that is 'different' and unknown. Although diabetes is covered in employment anti-discrimination laws, it is still of course possible for unprincipled employers to invent an excuse to make your role redundant or to make your position so unpleasant that you want to resign. Thankfully this is rare, and I would encourage you to tell your employer about your diabetes diagnosis. There are some circumstances in which you are obliged to inform your employer:

if your work involves operating machinery
if you are responsible for the welfare of others
if you are asked outright about your health.

What Does the Research Tell Us About the Experience of Diagnosis?

Kneck, Klang and Fagerberg (2011) interviewed individuals about their experience of being diagnosed, two months after diagnosis. Four themes emerged.

Taken over by a new reality

Previously familiar parts of life are now unknown and need renegotiating. Events such as travelling abroad, encountering a new challenge or getting a stomach infection suddenly demanded 'a new way of thinking'. Internal scripts and 'rules' of how to handle these events needed rewriting, which required psychological energy, investment and readjustment.

The body plays a role in life

A body that was familiar and knowable suddenly had new dimensions and demands. Unfamiliar and novel bodily symptoms (such as those signalling high or low blood sugar) increased awareness of the body, and new actions needed to be learned to manage it.

Different ways of learning

Obtaining, understanding and using information about diabetes felt complex and raised a number of questions. Uncertainty was a dominant feeling because of all the new situations and demands. New knowledge was required, but it also needed to be integrated with previous knowledge, which is mentally tiring.

The healthcare service as a necessary partner

The healthcare service was experienced as a rock to lean on, reliable and safe to turn to in case of uncertainty. However, this assumed that healthcare staff were accessible as well as being receptive to and focused on the needs of each individual. In practice, of course, this is challenging, and some participants were disappointed that there was only time to discuss concrete issues, such as doses and glucose levels, rather than their concerns and questions. Just as a child's caregiver enables him or her to grow in confidence by providing a safe base to return to when distressed, the healthcare service acted as the secure base to return to when participants needed explanations or wanted advice on how to act in different situations.

A diagnosis of diabetes is a significant life event. By becoming more mindful of how you are coping, and by taking steps to manage your experiences, you can allow diabetes to become an integrated part of your identity, which will enable you to work with it rather than fighting against it – essential for your health and wellbeing.

For the Healthcare Professional

It is difficult to tell someone that he or she has diabetes. Once you have delivered the facts, it can be challenging to know what to say in response to an emotional reaction. A stance of empathy without platitudes is advisable. There are some suggestions in the box below.

Helpful phrases for the newly diagnosed patient

'You have a right to feel upset about this.'

'This is a big life event and you will feel a whole range of feelings over the days to come.'

'Although these feelings might not feel normal to you, they are a normal response to receiving this news. They will ease with time.'

'This is hard.'

'This is a lot to take in.'

'Just as the diagnosis of diabetes lets us know there are physical changes happening in your body, receiving the diagnosis also causes emotional changes, and these can show themselves through tears, anger, being more short-tempered than usual, feeling more anxious and low in mood. This is normal.'

'It's OK to feel the way you do.'

'You have permission to feel upset/angry/scared about this.'

Unhelpful phrases

'This will get easier with time.'

'Things will get better.'

Trying to cheer the patient up.

What does the research tell us about diagnosis?

Although you might be wary about giving too much information at diagnosis in case of overwhelm, patients generally find more information helpful, particularly if they are advised to consume the material at a pace that suits their individual needs (Peel, Parry, Douglas and Lawton, 2004).

Polonsky, Fisher, Guzman et al. (2010) investigated both patients' experiences when they were diagnosed with type 2 diabetes and their diabetes-related distress and self-management five years after diagnosis. Current diabetes distress was significantly lower among those who reported that, at diagnosis, they had been reassured that diabetes could be managed successfully and instilled with a sense of hope, and had developed a clearer action plan with their healthcare professional.

Dietrich (1996) investigated attitudes of people with type 2 diabetes and found that the reaction and attitude physicians displayed towards a patient at the point of diagnosis was critical in influencing that patient's beliefs about the perceived seriousness of the disease and consequently their compliance. An inadequate perception of the seriousness of diabetes was a factor contributing to a lack of compliance.

The key points for the healthcare professional, then, are:

Give plenty of information about diabetes to take away. However, advise the person to use the material at their own pace.

Communicate that diabetes is a serious condition, while reassuring the patient that diabetes can be managed successfully.

Convey a sense of hope that they will learn to manage their condition with time.

Develop a clear action plan for the next steps – their next appointment, referral to a dietician, etc.

References

Becker, Gretchen (2004). *The First Year: Type 2 Diabetes*. Constable and Robinson, London.

Dietrich, U. (1996). Factors influencing the attitudes held by women with type II diabetes: a qualitative study. *Patient Education and Counseling*, 29(1), 13–23.

Edwards, Deborah (1987). Initial psychosocial impact of insulin-dependent diabetes mellitus on the pediatric client and family. *Issues in Comprehensive Pediatric Nursing*, 10(4), 196–207.

Fossum, M. and Mason, M. (1986). *Facing Shame: Families in Recovery*. W.W. Norton, London.

Greenberger, Dennis and Padesky, Christine (1995). *Mind Over Mood*. Guilford Press, New York.

Kneck, A., Klang, B. and Fagerberg, I. (2011). Learning to live with illness: experiences of persons with recent diagnoses of diabetes mellitus. *Scandinavian Journal of Caring Science*, 25(3), 558–66.

Kubler-Ross, E. (1997). *On Death and Dying*. Scribner Classics, New York.

Kubler-Ross, E. and Kessler, D. (2005). *On Grief and Grieving*. Scribner, New York.

Peel, E., Parry, O., Douglas, M. and Lawton, J. (2004). Diagnosis of type 2 diabetes: a qualitative analysis of patients' emotional reactions and views about information provision. *Patient Education and Counseling*, 53(3), 269–75.

Polonsky, William (1999). *Diabetes Burnout*. American Diabetes Association. Alexandria, VA.

Polonsky, W., Fisher, L., Guzman, S., Sieber, W., Philis-Tsimikas, A. and Edelman, S. (2010). Are patients' initial experiences at the diagnosis of type 2 diabetes associated with attitudes and self-management over time? *Diabetes Educator*, 36(5), 828–34.

Rubin, A. and Jarvis, S. (2007). *Diabetes for Dummies*. Wiley-Blackwell, Chichester.

Further Reading

Gretchen Becker (2004). *The First Year, Type 2 Diabetes*. Constable and Robinson, London.

Dennis Greenberger and Christine Padesky (1995). *Mind Over Mood*. Guilford Press, New York.

E. Kubler-Ross and D. Kessler (2005). *On Grief and Grieving*. Scribner, New York.

William Polonsky (1999). *Diabetes Burnout*. American Diabetes Association, Alexandria, VA.

J. Rogers and R. Walker (2006). *Type 2 Diabetes: Your Questions Answered*. Dorling Kindersley, London.

J. Rogers and R. Walker (2010). *Diabetes: A Practical Guide to Managing your Health*. Dorling Kindersley, London.

A. Rubin and S. Jarvis (2007). *Diabetes for Dummies*. Wiley-Blackwell, Chichester.

4

Depression, Low Mood and Burnout

The link between diabetes and depression was recognized as far back as the seventeenth century, when the English physician Thomas Willis observed in 1674 that diabetes often manifested in patients who had experienced significant sadness, life stress or a long period of anguish. Research demonstrates that at least one third of people with diabetes have a lifetime risk of developing depression (Ali, Stone, Peters et al., 2006; Barnard, Skinner and Peveler, 2006). Some studies have shown that lower levels of depressive symptoms are common in 31–45% of people with diabetes (Gary, Crum, Cooper-Patrick et al., 2000; Hermanns, Kulzer, Krichbaum et al., 2005). The burden of diabetes care, with its necessary lifestyle changes and unremitting self-management tasks, detrimentally affects the quality of life of the person with diabetes (Rubin, 2000). We know that individuals with diabetes who struggle with low mood do not fare as well, in terms of the severity of their symptoms, complications and general wellbeing, as those whose mood remains high. (Ciechanowksi, Katon and Russon, 2000). Diabetes 'burnout', a distinct yet related issue, is also common for people who have been managing diabetes over a long period of time (Polonsky, Anderson, Lohrer et al., 1995). This chapter aims to describe depression, burnout, and their symptoms, explore the reasons why difficulties with mood can develop, and describe strategies for managing and overcoming depression.

Diabetes and Wellbeing: Managing the Psychological and Emotional Challenges of Diabetes Types 1 and 2, First Edition. Dr Jen Nash.
© 2013 John Wiley & Sons, Ltd. Published 2013 by John Wiley & Sons, Ltd.

What is Depression?

According to the World Health Organization, 'Depression is a common mental disorder that presents with depressed mood, loss of interest or pleasure, feelings of guilt or low self-worth, disturbed sleep or appetite, low energy, and poor concentration. These problems can become chronic or recurrent and lead to substantial impairments in an individual's ability to take care of his or her everyday responsibilities. At its worst, depression can lead to suicide, a tragic fatality associated with the loss of about 850 000 lives every year' (World Health Organization, 2012).

People with diabetes are two to three times more likely to be considered depressed than those without diabetes (Pouwer, Geelhoed-Duijveestihn, Tack et al., 2010). Further, the diabetes–depression link is bi-directional, meaning that not only do those living with diabetes often manifest depression, but people with depression are more vulnerable to the development of type 2 diabetes (Mezuk, Eaton, Albrecht and Golden, 2008; Pouwer, Beekman and Nijpels, 2003). Research has attempted to ascertain whether depression increases the risk of type 1 diabetes, but it is still unclear, with studies yielding very mixed results (Barnard, Skinner and Peveler, 2006).

This is grim reading, and I am afraid it does not stop there. In addition to those individuals who meet the diagnostic criteria for depression, many people (both with and without diabetes) are living with what is termed 'non-clinical' depression. This describes symptoms of low mood that do not reach a level at which depression would be diagnosable, but still experience a marked decrease in quality of life (Gary, Crum, Cooper-Patrick et al., 2000; Hermanns, Kulzer, Krichbaum et al., 2005). Furthermore, still others are struggling with 'burnout', a linked yet distinct form of low mood specific to those with diabetes (Polonsky, Anderson, Lohrer et al., 1995). Although the research paints a bleak picture, the good news is that depression and diabetes-related burnout are treatable, and many people go on to make a full recovery. The other good news (although it might be little comfort if you are in the midst of dealing with depression right now) is that many people who recover from depression report that the experience deepened their self-knowledge and understanding of life. This has aided them in other respects, helping them to become more self-aware, more sensitive to others and more thoughtful as parents, for example.

Why Does Depression Occur?

Most practitioners agree that there is not one specific cause of depression. Rather it is viewed from a 'biopsychosocial' perspective: biological, psychological and social factors contribute to its development.

Biological factors

Some people are more susceptible to developing depression than others. Those with close relatives who have been diagnosed with depression (especially parents or siblings) are more at risk. Further, there are also individual differences in the biochemical make-up of the human brain. Two brain chemicals, noradrenaline and serotonin, play an important role in the transmission of nerve impulses within the brain, and these can be deficient in people with depression. There is also emerging evidence that biological mechanisms, such as overactivity in the hypothalamic-pituitary-adrenal axis, may explain the depression–type 2 diabetes link (Ismail, 2010).

The biological aspect of your mood regulation is therefore outside your voluntary control, in the same way as when you catch a cold or flu. It can be helpful to view your depression in this way, and treat yourself kindly just as you would if you had a physical ailment (Butler and Hope, 1995).

Psychological factors

There are psychological factors that contribute to the development of depression. In addition to unhelpful thinking styles, which we will focus on later in this chapter, many psychologists view depression as a natural reaction to loss. As we discussed in chapter 3, the diagnosis of diabetes can often lead to a sense of loss, similar to that experienced in the grieving process. Loss of status, hope or self-image is the key problematic area, and each of these can be relevant for the person with diabetes. Loss of status can be felt when a person loses a valued role, such as being the 'healthy' one in the family. Loss of self-image can occur with the realization that you are not 100 per cent fit and healthy. Hope can be lost by many with diabetes who feel that their diabetes is in control of them, rather than vice versa. Depression can also be a mask for anger. As we learned in chapter 3, anger can also be a natural reaction to diagnosis, but it is often viewed as a socially unacceptable emotion to express. Depression can mask the patient's anger towards diabetes; he or she directs the bad feelings towards diabetes at the self.

Social factors

Social factors are also important in the development of depression. Family and work stresses, feeling lonely and isolated, loss of a loved one, a major life event such as an accident, loss of job or illness in the family, are all things that make us feel less in control of our lives. If bad things can happen out of the blue like this, you can feel powerless and that your actions don't matter.

Further, you may be actually gaining a payoff from your depression. It may seem punishing to suggest this but Rowe (2003), a psychologist who herself has suffered with depression, speaks very frankly of the possible payoffs of experiencing periods of low mood. For instance, depression can allow you to avoid some things you may be scared of, such as facing responsibilities or carrying out duties (in your work or family role), that you find stressful or overwhelming. It can also serve to obstruct your need to make uncertain and frightening changes in your life, such as leaving a partner, or standing up to someone who is bullying you. Depression, therefore, rather than being the problem, can be a *symptom* of an underlying difficulty that really needs to be faced. As long as the problem remains unresolved, the depression continues. Depression can therefore be reformulated as a fear of change, allowing you to stay stuck in the current, albeit unpleasant, crucially *knowable* place where you are. As you read this chapter, if you find yourself responding, 'yes but...' (Rowe, 2003) to suggestions that might help you, either those that follow in this chapter, or the advice of those around you; in that case I encourage you to be curious about whether there could be a hidden payoff to your depression.

How is Depression Diagnosed?

Depression is diagnosed by examining your depressive symptoms over the past two weeks. This can be done either in conversation with your healthcare professional or by completing a written questionnaire. The symptoms are described in a set of diagnostic criteria in the Diagnostic and Statistical Manual (American Psychiatric Association, 2000). If you think you may be currently suffering from depression, you are likely to notice changes in your bodily symptoms, thinking, emotions and behaviour. Here are the most commonly reported signs and symptoms of depression (Butler and Hope, 1995)

Thinking

Inability to concentrate
Inability to make decisions
Loss of interest in the things going on around you, and in other people
Self-criticism: 'I've made a mess of everything'
Self-blame: 'It's all my fault'
Self-loathing: 'I'm utterly useless'
Activities seem pointless
Pessimism: 'This will never change', 'There's nothing I can do'
Preoccupation with problems, failures and bad feelings
Believing you deserve to be punished
Thinking about harming yourself

Feelings

Sadness, misery, unhappiness
Feeling overwhelmed by everyday demands, feeling burdened
Low confidence and poor self-esteem
Loss of pleasure, satisfaction and enjoyment
Apathy, numbness
Feeling disappointed, discouraged or hopeless
Feeling unattractive or ugly
Helplessness
Irritability, tension, anxiety and worry
Guilt

Behaviour

Reduced activity levels; doing less than usual
Everything feels like an effort
Difficulty getting out of bed in the morning
Withdrawal – from people, work, relaxations or pleasures
Bouts of restlessness
Sighing, groaning, crying

Bodily changes

Loss of appetite, or increased appetite
Disturbed sleep, especially waking early in the morning
Loss of interest in sex
Fatigue, lack of energy, or exhaustion
Inertia: inability to get going, dragging oneself around

Assessing your symptoms of depression

In order to gain insight into your current level of depression, take a minute now to complete the Patient Health Questionnaire-9 (Kroenke, Spitzer and Williams, 2001), a self-report questionnaire that is commonly used in clinical practice.

What have you discovered? Perhaps you are not currently experiencing many (or any) depressive symptoms at all, in which you can move ahead to another chapter, or read the information that follows as a reference in case your mood changes in the future. Alternatively, you may be at the other extreme, and your score demonstrates that you are struggling with significant depression currently. If so, the following sections will help you to understand why you are feeling this way and how to start right away to make improvements to your mood.

Before that, though, it is important that I advise you if you have responded positively to question 9 of the PHQ-9. If you have been experiencing thoughts that you would be better off dead or of hurting yourself in some way, it is essential that you take these thoughts seriously. You are not 'going mad'. Many people, with and without diabetes, have times in their life when things have felt difficult to cope with, and have considered self-harm or taking their own life. Some reports suggest that one in six people have thought about suicide (although the incidence may actually be higher, as some people may not want to admit it). Turn to the end of this chapter for specific advice for severe depression.

Diabetes and Depression

Depression has been found to be approximately two to three times more common in patients with a chronic physical health problem (such as cancer, heart disease or diabetes) than in people who have good physical health

Table 4.1   Patient Health Questionnaire 9 (Kroenke, Spitzer and Williams, 2001)

Over the last two weeks, how often have you been bothered by any of the following problems?

	Not at All	*On Several Days*	*On More than Half the Days*	*Nearly Every Day*
1. Little interest or pleasure in doing things				
2. Feeling down, depressed, or hopeless				
3. Trouble falling/staying asleep, sleeping too much				
4. Feeling tired or having little energy				
5. Poor appetite or overeating				
6. Feeling bad about yourself, or that you are a failure or have let yourself or your family down				
7. Trouble concentrating on things, such as reading the newspaper or watching television.				
8. Moving or speaking so slowly that other people could have noticed. Or the opposite – being so fidgety or restless that you have been moving around a lot more than usual.				
9. Thoughts that you would be better off dead or of hurting yourself in some way.				

Score your answers in the following way:

Not at all	0
On several days	1
On more than half the days	2
Nearly every day	3

Now look at your totals.

1–4	Minimal depression
5–9	Mild depression
10–14	Moderate depression
15–19	Moderately severe depression
20–27	Severe depression

(National Institute for Health and Clinical Excellence, 2011). Diabetes is a chronic illness that involves a high degree of self-care tasks and is a demanding condition to manage. Diabetes and depression often interact with each other, exacerbating the downward spiral of mood. For example:

You feel low in mood.
You aren't as motivated to care for your diabetes.
Your diabetes self-care is poorer.
Your blood glucose levels become higher.
You experience greater fatigue and lethargy.
You feel lower in mood, even less motivated to care for diabetes, and so on.

Depression is more common in patients with diabetes who are female, live alone, have experienced late or acute complications and have experienced a critical life event in the past or had poor glycaemic control (Hermanns, Kulzer, Krichbaum, Kubiak and Haak, 2006).

Depression or diabetes burnout?

Subclinical depression is the term used to describe individuals who present with depressive symptoms but do not meet the criteria for a diagnosis of clinical depression. Approximately one third of people with type 1 diabetes and 37–43% of people with type 2 diabetes in the Netherlands reported significant symptoms of low mood but were not diagnosed with clinical depression (Pouwer and Hermanns, 2009). Individuals with subclinical depression are particularly at risk as they do not qualify for referral for treatment and have to suffer with their symptoms alone.

There are also a significant number of individuals who do not report symptoms of depression, but still feel low in relation to their diabetes. These individuals may be struggling with diabetes-specific distress, coined diabetes 'burnout' (Polonsky, 1999) Diabetes burnout occurs when a person feels 'overwhelmed by diabetes and the frustrating burden of diabetes self-care' (Polonsky, 1999). These emotions may be very different to feelings of depression. However, they can still be very destructive and have serious implications for care.

Symptoms of burnout include (Barnard, Lloyd and Holt, 2012):

Feeling overwhelmed and defeated by diabetes
Feeling angry about diabetes, frustrated by the self-care regime and/or having strong negative feelings about diabetes
Feeling that diabetes is controlling their life

Worrying about not taking care of diabetes well enough, yet unable, unmotivated or unwilling to change
Avoiding diabetes-related tasks that might give feedback about the consequences of poor control
Feeling alone and isolated with diabetes.

As you can see, diabetes burnout centres on feelings focused specifically on diabetes, while depression affects the person in broader psychological ways in which the person has negative thoughts about the self and the world, and a hopelessness about the future. The strategies that follow can be helpful whether you are experiencing depression or diabetes burnout.

How to Manage Depression

Just as there are biological, psychological and social causes of depression, treatment can also be addressed at these levels. Antidepressant medication, changing daily activities, adapting unhelpful thinking styles and being thoughtful about available support systems are all possible biological, psychological and social routes to alleviating depression and low mood.

Antidepressant medications

Antidepressant medications containing the brain chemicals that may be in short supply in those with depression can sometimes be helpful in treating moderate to severe depression, in the same way that insulin is lacking and needs to be externally administered in type 1 diabetes. Antidepressants can cause side effects for some people, and the type and dose need careful management by your GP or other prescribing clinician. As antidepressants only work at the biological level and not the psychological or social levels, they are ideally taken in conjunction with psychological and social strategies for overcoming depression. Antidepressants can help those who are feeling very low to raise their mood enough to feel less overwhelmed and more able to engage in active, change-oriented coping strategies, such as increasing activities, altering thinking styles and gaining support.

Increase your activities

Depression robs you of your energy, so the tasks that you could previously do without thinking now feel overwhelming. Just as when you have a cold or flu you do not have the energy to get the jobs of life done, depression interferes with your ability to achieve even the most straightforward tasks of life. When you are considering increasing your activities, it is important to focus on one change at a time. Don't think you have to get it all done at once. Depression causes undermining and bleak thoughts such as, 'It won't make any difference', 'There's no point in trying' and 'It all feels like too much for me to bother'. Instead, shift your focus from the destination just to the next small step on the journey to getting better. You won't feel completely better all at once, so don't try to. Just aim for feeling a little better today, and the rest will take care of itself.

Think about some of the everyday tasks that you are struggling with at the moment and write them in the space below. Here are some ideas of everyday undertakings that many people with depression find difficult:

Getting dressed in the morning
Having a shower
Making a phone call
Collecting your children from school
Shopping
Laundry
Ironing
Writing a letter or email
Meeting up with a friend
Responding to bills

Activities I am struggling with at the moment:

_____

_____

_____

_____

_____

_____

_____

_____

_____

_____

Step 1: Diary of daily activities   Now you have a list of tasks that you find difficult, you can begin to find out how to tackle them. Beck (1970), who you may remember from Chapter 2 as the founder of CBT, strongly recommended keeping a diary of daily activities. It is such an effective component of improving depression that it is still commonly advised as an ideal starting point. Part of the difficulty with depression is that you may find yourself thinking back over the day and believing that you did not do or achieve anything. Keeping a simple diary provides you with evidence that you did indeed accomplish something, and shifts your focus so that you can see this more clearly.

There are four stages to keeping the diary, but don't let this overwhelm you: just start with the first step and only move on to step 2 when you have got a comfortable grasp of the previous one.

Look at the example activity diary. Each hour of your waking day has a slot for you to fill in everything that you do. Have the diary somewhere you will see it throughout the day to remind you to complete it. Once you have completed one day successfully, congratulate yourself. This is itself an achievement and a significant step on your road to recovery. Continue filling out the diary in the same way the next day and move on to step 2 when you feel ready.

Step 2: Give each activity a rating   To feel good about our lives, we must experience two aspects to our activities: pleasure and mastery (which is another word for achievement). If you are depressed, both of these essential elements of life are at risk: depression means you are prone to feeling like you don't want to engage in the activities that give you pleasure – and tasks that involve a certain level of mastery or achievement tend to feel difficult to do – even if ordinarily you find them very easy. Step 2 is to look over your activity diary and score each for its level of challenge. Score the activity on a scale of 0–10, where 0 is no difficulty at all and 10 is the most difficult task you could imagine doing. Remember that these ratings relate to how difficult you find them *at the moment*, not at a time in the past when you may have felt more capable. While ordinarily you might pick up the phone at work to call a customer with no hesitation, this is just the sort of task that is apt to feel more challenging now you are struggling with depression. Give yourself a 'mastery' rating (independent of how you might have performed on the call – this rating just relates to the sheer fact you did it). So if you score yourself a 7 for this task, write M=7 to signify this on your diary. Do not spend time wrestling too much between ratings (e.g. 'Am I a 6 or a 7?'). Just go for the figure that feels most appropriate.

Table 4.2   Example activity diary

Time	Friday	Saturday	Sunday
6–7am	Awake in bed	Asleep	
7–8	Shower	Asleep	
8–9	Commute to work	Breakfast	
9–10	Emails	Watched TV	
10–11	Meeting with boss	Went to the park	
11–12	Report writing	Shopping	
12–1pm	Phone calls	Lunch with sister	
1–2	Lunch at desk	Lunch with sister	
2–3	Meeting	Internet	
3–4	Typed up minutes	Housework	
4–5	Emails	Housework	
5–6	Commute home	Coffee & phone call	
6–7	Phone call – mum	TV	
7–8	Dinner	Dinner at home	
8–9	TV	Drinks with friend	
9–10	TV	Cinema	
10–11	Chores	Cinema	
11–12	Read book	Home, read book	
12–1am	Sleep	Sleep	

Next, go through your diary a second time, and rate the activities in terms of pleasure. Again, give each one a rating. A score of 0 signifies no pleasure at all, while a 10 signifies immense pleasure. Mark your diary again. For example, if you gave playing with your children a pleasure rating of 5, mark P=5 beside this activity.

Step 3: Get curious   Now you are aware of the extent of pleasure and mastery in your life, the third step is to get curious about how you spend your time in the week and how you can increase the pleasure and mastery

Table 4.3 Activity diary

Time	Mon	Tues	Wed	Thur	Fri	Sat	Sun
6–7am							
7–8							
8–9							
9–10							
10–11							
11–12							
12–1pm							
1–2							
2–3							
3–4							
4–5							
5–6							
6–7							
7–8							
8–9							
9–10							
10–11							
11–12							
12–1am							

aspects each day. Review your activity diary and ask yourself the following questions (Greenberger and Padesky, 1995):

1. Did my mood change during the week? How? What patterns do I notice?
2. Did my activities affect my mood? How?
3. What activities helped me feel better? Why? Are these activities in my best long-term interest? What other activities could I do that might also make me feel better?

4. What activities made me feel worse? Why? Are these activities in my best interest?
5. Were there certain times of the day (e.g. mornings) or week (e.g. weekends) when I felt worse?
6. Can I think of anything I could do to feel better during these times?
7. Were there certain times of the day or week when I felt better?
8. Looking at my answers to questions 3 and 4, what activities can I plan in the coming week to increase the chances that I will feel better this week? Over the next few months?

Here are some further specific questions about mastery and pleasure (Butler and Hope, 1995).

Questions to ask yourself about mastery

How do I feel if I make no effort to do the things that are difficult?
How do I feel if I do them, and give myself credit for doing them?
Which are the major trouble spots in my day?
What could I do to make it easier to master these difficult times?

Questions to ask yourself about pleasure

What things are most enjoyable at the moment?
How could I do more of these things?
What could I do to increase the amount of pleasure I have each day?
What sorts of things used to give me pleasure?
Are there things I have stopped doing that I used to enjoy?

Step 4: Make a plan   Use the questions you have answered in the previous steps to make a plan for the coming week.

Plan more fun   It is important to treat yourself to enough fun in life. Many areas of life can feel like hard work and chores when you are feeling depressed, so duties and recreation need to be appropriately balanced. Devising a routine that incorporates pleasure into your day can be useful: for example, deciding that you will do something enjoyable in the hour or 30 minutes before you start preparing/eating lunch or dinner each day. Take a look at the suggestions below for some ideas of how you can incorporate more fun into your life (Butler and Hope, 1995).

Category	Examples
Relaxation	Listening to music, taking a long bath, calling a friend, reading a novel or magazine, sitting by the fire, or in the garden or park (depending on the weather!)
Activities	Taking a walk, watching TV or a video, planning an outing, enjoying a hobby, doing a puzzle or the crossword, playing bridge, poker, solitaire, or your favourite game of cards with friends, gardening, going to a coffee shop or a restaurant for dinner
Things to eat or drink	Having your favourite meal, a tea or coffee, a new piece of fruit
Treats	Buying a bunch of flowers or a bar of scented soap or handcream, planning a trip to the theatre, buying a new piece of clothing, getting up late
Time	Ten minutes on your own, a mid-morning break, a proper lunch hour, time to think, a weekend break, a holiday
Exercise	Joining the local gym, taking an exercise class, going for a swim, walking the dog
Self-talk	I'm doing fine, I'm really pleased with . . . , Well done, you can make it, you deserve a break
Setting limits	Number of chores, bedtime, a time to stop work, demands made by others
Other people	Chatting on the phone with or visiting a friend or relative, having a long lunch with an old friend.

Plan more absorbing activities   Activities that demand attention are good as they distract you from thoughts that may make your mood worse. Watching a film, reading a book or magazine or engaging in a hobby or craft can all be engrossing choices.

Plan more pursuits that raise your energy level   Moving your body each day actually raises your energy. We all need a certain amount of daily activity and movement to avoid lethargy – the less you do the more tired you feel. Schedule activities that require movement or gentle exercise: taking the dog (yours or a neighbour's) for a walk, gardening, housework or walking to the local shop.

Continue to complete your activity diary for another week and then ask yourself the eight review questions (above) again and see what changes you notice.

Your Thoughts: Using CBT to Overcome Depression

As you discovered in chapter 2, there is a very close relationship between the emotions you are experiencing and the way you are thinking. When you are feeling low, your thoughts and memories will tend to be more negative. You are more likely to remember the bad things that have happened. This makes your mood more downbeat, which causes your thoughts to deteriorate further, and so on, until a downward spiral of increasing depression is established.

The downward spiral of depressed mood

I *think* of what is wrong with my life (thought)
I *feel* sad, disappointed, upset, angry, frustrated (feeling)
I blame myself for all my faults and problems (thought)
I feel more depressed (feeling)
I can't see a way out (thought)
I feel hopeless (feeling)

Using CBT strategies intervenes in this downward spiral by changing some of these negative patterns of thinking. As your habitual thinking styles start to get more positive, the depressed moods start to improve, which gives you impetus for more positive thoughts and feelings until the spiral is halted and reversed.

Thoughts that are common to depression

Below is a list of thoughts that are very commonplace for people struggling with depression. Review this list and see how many are familiar to you. By realizing that your thoughts are not unique to you, you can see that they may be the depression talking, rather than individual to you and your situation.

I feel like I'm up against the world
I'm no good

Why can't I ever succeed?
No one understands me
I've let myself down
I've let other people down
I don't think I can go on
I wish I were a better person
I'm so weak
I'm useless
My life's not going the way I want it to
I'm so disappointed in myself
Nothing feels good any more
I can't get started
I can't get motivated
What's wrong with me?
I wish I were somewhere else
I can't get things together
I hate myself
I'm worthless
I wish I could just disappear
What's the matter with me?
I'm a loser
My life is a mess
I'm a failure
I'll never make it
I feel so helpless
Something has to change
There must be something wrong with me
My future is bleak
Life is pointless
It's just not worth it
I can't finish anything

When you are depressed and experience these powerful thoughts, it is as if they are telling the truth about you and your life. They feel immensely personal, but the reality is that virtually all people with depression will read these thoughts and identify with them. In the same way as physical conditions have symptoms (e.g. thirst and excessive urination in diabetes), emotional difficulties also have symptoms. Thoughts of this nature are one of the symptoms of depression.

Let's look at a case study to help us see how CBT can be used to tackle negative thoughts.

Case study: Helen

Helen is 54 and has had type 2 diabetes for 10 years. She has been struggling recently with stress at work as there has been lots of talk of redundancies, and she has also been spending more time caring for her mother, who has dementia. She has felt less motivated to do things lately and the exercise routine she had established in the years following diagnosis has fallen by the wayside. She also finds herself eating more sweet and unhealthy food to try and cheer herself up when she's watching TV on the sofa in the evening. As a result she missed her last diabetes health check and has not rescheduled one as she is scared she will get told off for letting the weight she had lost creep back on. She was shocked to discover that her scores on the PHQ-9 revealed that she is struggling with depression. She knew she had been feeling quite low, but had not realized that the changes to her sleep, appetite and concentration were also signs of depression. She was also surprised to realize that she felt a little relieved. Understanding that she was not going 'mad' and that lots of people with diabetes struggle with feeling low at times was reassuring. She could see that, by working through the steps in this chapter, she could start to make some changes. She felt uncertain about whether to talk to her GP or diabetes care team about a referral for professional support. She decided she would first talk to a cousin of hers, whose husband had struggled with depression a few years earlier. Helen's 5-step thought-challenging process looks like this.

Step 1: What is the situation or event?

Lying awake in bed in the morning
Getting home after work
Watching TV on the sofa in the evening
Shopping
Putting the phone down after a conversation with a family member about
Mum's dementia

Step 2: What do you tell yourself? What are the thoughts you notice running through your mind?

I'm no good
My life is a mess
There's nothing I can do to change this
I'm all on my own
I'm useless
I should be able to cope better than this
I hate myself
There must be something wrong with me

Step 3: What is happening in your body and what do you do?

Mood – low, depressed, sad, lonely, tense, worried, upset, confused, miserable
Body sensations – feeling heavy, muscle tension
Behaviours – doing less of the activities I previously enjoyed, staying in bed later in the morning, eating more food.

Step 4: Challenge your thoughts by asking yourself some helpful questions

What is the evidence for and against this thought?
Is thinking this way helping me?
Are there other ways of thinking about this situation?
If a friend told me they were thinking this way, how would I respond?
Am I thinking in 'all or nothing' terms?
What other points of view are there?
How would someone else think about this?
How else could I think about it?
How would I think about this if I were feeling better?
What are the facts of the case?
How can I find out which way of thinking fits the facts best?
What is the evidence?
Could I be making a mistake in the way I am thinking?

Am I thinking straight?

Am I pressurizing myself?

Am I using the language of the extremist?

What is the worst think that could happen?

How bad is this going to get?

What can I do when that happens?

How can I get help?

Step 5: Come up with an alternative, balanced thought

'My whole life is a mess.' I've still got a job and a roof over my head. Yes, I feel a bit of a mess, and the house is a bit of a mess, but I've still got my family and my dog. I've felt a bit of a mess at other times in my life, and got through them.

'There's nothing I can do to change this.' The word nothing is very extreme. I could talk to someone about what I'm worrying about and see if they have any ideas for things I could do to change the situation. I could plan something enjoyable to balance out the chores of life.

'I'm all on my own.' It is true, I am sitting her on my own right now, but I'm not completely alone in the world. I have [inserts names of friend, family member, colleague, neighbour]. I have made friends before, so I can probably make new ones too. I could go to a Diabetes Support Group and meet some new people there.

'I'm useless.' If a friend said that to me, I would be really offended. I know it is not true and saying it to myself only makes me feel worse. Yes, I have made some mistakes in my life, but that does not mean I am useless. It is a complete exaggeration.

'I should be able to cope better than this.' I am should-ing on myself again! It really puts the pressure on. Maybe lots of people going through what I am right now would struggle. I am coping in some ways [insert the facts: I've got a roof over my head, my children love me, I'm learning new things at work, and about my health through reading this book. Although I feel depressed, it doesn't make me less of a person. Although I do not like feeling this way, it will pass. Every time I think of new ways to think about my situation, I am getting better.

Distraction   When depressed, you may find that you often get caught up in intellectualizing and analysing the thoughts that occur in low mood. Actually, thoughts are just thoughts. Distraction can help shift your attention on to new thoughts that are more helpful to you.

Negative thinking needs interrupting. Because the processing capacity of our brain is limited, we can only think a certain number of thoughts at one time. When you are feeling depressed, your default is to think about negative things. The quickest way to interrupt these default thoughts is to use distraction. Involve yourself in an absorbing activity, preferably one that involves using your hands, not just your mind – like using your computer, doing a crossword or Sudoku puzzle, organizing a drawer or desk, sewing, knitting, fixing something, trimming your nails, tidying up, gardening, sorting your recycling, writing a shopping list. Activities also provide us with the opportunity to succeed at something or get something done.

Use your mouth and your brain – by singing a song, humming a jingle from an advert, talking to someone else, or speaking aloud a poem or prayer that you might know.

Do something pleasurable – have a relaxing bath, talk with someone you like, buy yourself a small treat like a magazine or your favourite coffee, read a book, watch a funny film. See the 'Plan more fun' section earlier on in the chapter for more ideas of enjoyable activities.

Play counting games – such as how many dog walkers or blue cars you can notice, or count backwards from 100 in 3's, or multiply by 7's.

Describe an object – this shifts your attention outside yourself and into the world. Choose an object in your immediate surroundings. Pretend you had to describe it in precise detail to an alien who had never seen it before. What is its colour, shape, function, texture?

Use a sensory awareness exercise – become conscious of what you can hear right now – the hum of the refrigerator, birds outside the window, the tapping of your partner at their computer keyboard. Then shift your awareness to what you can feel – the sensation of your legs and back against the chair, the feeling of your clothes on your skin, the impression of this book in your hands. In the same way, what can you see and smell?

Getting Support

A number of studies have shown that having the benefit of support through a close, confiding relationship is an incredibly powerful protection against developing depression. Do try and reach out to someone you trust about what you are going through. You may be embarrassed, or feel that depression is your fault, or that there is something wrong with you. There may be stigma in your culture for any signs of emotional vulnerability and you may not want to worry others with your problems.

It may feel hard to risk opening up, you may not want to worry those you love, and you might fear that talking about these thoughts may make them worse. Actually, the reverse is true: talking about troubling thoughts won't make them worse and usually brings some relief. Those you love can probably sense that you aren't quite yourself anyway, and so sharing what's going on and letting them be there for you is helpful to them and allows them to feel there is something they can do to support you.

Talking with someone can assist you to think about your problems in a new way, help you solve them and offer a different perspective. Knowing that you have the support of someone who cares is helpful. They can help you to stay on track with commitments you have decided to make to help you through it, such as keeping an activity log or doing the other exercises in this chapter.

A good first step could be to put your thoughts and feelings to paper and write down what you might say, either in the form of a diary or journal or as a letter. You could then share this with your loved one. However, even if you decide not to share what you have written with anyone, there is good evidence that simply writing down your thoughts and feelings can have a positive influence on your mood (Blair, 2008). Rather than your thoughts spinning around out of control inside your head, it can show you that they do in fact have a beginning and an end. This can help you feel more in control of them, and your feelings.

Seeking support from a professional

You may not have anyone in your life that you feel able to talk to about your depression. Sometimes your loved one can be too close to your problems, or too much a part of them, to be the ideal person to help you. A psychologist, counsellor or therapist can fill the dual role of someone to help you solve problems and an individual to be accountable to for the changes that might feel challenging but that ultimately you need to make in order to get better. Seeing the upcoming appointment with your psychologist in your diary and remembering that you have yet to phone an old friend you agreed to connect with may provide that much-needed impetus you need to pick up the phone and move forward.

Accepting professional help in the form of counselling or therapy does not mean that you are 'crazy' or 'mad'. There is, unfortunately, still a lot of stigma associated with seeking help from a therapist (an umbrella term for various helping professionals including psychologists, counsellors, psychotherapists, psychoanalysts and psychiatrists). An old-fashioned view still prevails that we must keep a 'stiff upper lip' about any problems that are emotional in nature. Again, the reverse is true. It takes much inner courage, strength and bravery to confront and deal with personal vulnerabilities in the therapy room. Stereotypes prevail about what a counselling relationship involves. While some people in some types of therapy do lie on the couch talking about their relationship with their mother or father, the large majority do not! Rather, they use action-oriented strategies based around problems in the here and now, and while attention can be turned to early experiences and relationships if that's helpful, there is much that can be done that relates to the material in the present. As you will see from the material in this book, CBT is very much about your thoughts, emotions and behaviours in the here and now.

As with any relationship in life, you will 'click' with some therapists' styles more than others. Do not despair then if you had an experience previously in which you didn't really feel a connection to a therapist. Most therapists will suggest that you have an initial consultation to get a sense of how working together over a longer duration may be. Therapy duration varies. Relief normally starts at the first session, and for some people only a small number of sessions (3–6) are needed to gain benefit (NICE guidelines recommend 6–8 sessions for moderate depression with a chronic health problem, increasing to 16–18 sessions for severe depression). Look at the recommended resources at the end of this chapter for ideas on how to find a therapist.

Special Advice for Severe Depression

If you are very depressed, the recommendations in this chapter may feel too overwhelming and complex for you. Listed below are the essentials to focus on. Start here and come back to this chapter when you are feeling stronger and more able to implement the other strategies.

Seek professional help

Don't struggle alone. Avenues of support include psychological therapy, medication, or both, as described above. See your GP or diabetes healthcare professional, who will be able to advise you on referral options in your local area. For non-NHS sores of support, see the Further Reading section at the end of the chapter.

Give yourself praise for the simple tasks you are achieving

When you are very depressed the everyday tasks of life, such as getting up in the morning, having a shower, getting dressed and preparing meals, can feel like very hard work. It is important to divide big tasks into smaller segments. Everyday responsibilities that feel overwhelming need to be broken down and focused on one piece at a time. Compared with your usual standards when feeling good, it might seem a little pathetic to operate in this way. But would you blame someone who had a broken leg for not being able to go for their usual exercise routine? When you are depressed, everything feels like more of an effort. Your goals need to be smaller to ensure you succeed, and doing something (rather than nothing) is the most important thing.

So if getting out of bed to start the day feels too much, simply focus on the first part of this task:

'I just need to swing my feet out of bed and place them on the floor.'
Once this is achieved, encourage yourself. 'Well done – that's the hardest
    part done! Now I just need to lift my weight on to my feet and stand up.'
'Good work. Now I'm standing I'm going to have a stretch. If I notice a
    thought telling me to get back into bed, I'm going to remind myself that
    if I still feel this way in 20 minutes, I have permission to return to bed.'
'Excellent. Now I'm going to head to the bathroom and use the loo.'
'That feels better. OK, now I'm going to turn the shower on. It will be good
    to feel the hot water on my skin.'
And so on . . . .

The most important message is, Don't try to do too much. Go easy on yourself. The kinder and more compassionate you can be, the quicker you will get back to your usual self and your usual level of activity.

Special Advice if You are Feeling Suicidal

Firstly, if you feel a strong desire to act on thoughts that you might harm yourself, or are making plans to, it is crucial that you seek help at once. If it feels impossible to reach out to a family member, friend or health professional directly, then do call the Samaritans, where someone is available to listen and support you 24 hours a day (see the number at the end of this chapter). Also, know that all hospital Accident & Emergency departments are open throughout the day and night, and provide access to mental health professionals who can offer you care and support while you are feeling vulnerable.

If the suicidal feelings are less well formed and more of a desire to escape the overwhelming sense of things being too much to deal with right now, then think about the following questions:

What would prevent me from acting on this feeling?
If I get through this and the depression lifts, what would I like to be able to do in the future?
Are any of my problems so unsolvable that no solution could ever be found?

Remember that these low thoughts are your depression talking. Others who have had times in their life in which they felt suicidal but didn't act on those thoughts categorically report that they are grateful they never acted on these feelings. No matter how bad and bleak life felt at that time, lighter days always came along and life became worth living and fighting for again.

Supporting a Loved One Who is Depressed

If a loved one has depression, any support you can provide them is invaluable. This can be challenging, though. You can see they are not themselves, and want to offer them sympathy and support, but often your reasonable suggestions are rejected or ignored, which can be irritating and frustrating. Remember that your loved one is not themselves; you may not like them very much at times.

Maintain confidentiality at all times. It is important that the person who is depressed can trust you not to share information they are telling you with others. Although you are not a counsellor, you can feel more equipped by being aware of the basic principles of counselling skills. You are not to solve other people's problems for them, or to give advice (unless it is directly asked for; and even then encourage independence). Rather, your main objective is to listen and then reflect back what you have understood. Hearing their experience voiced can help the person with low mood to see their situation more clearly and perhaps see the different options that might be available to them, or even just the next step. You can be active to listen out for 'change talk' and encourage them to decide what specific goal they will set themselves (e.g. phone the nurse on Tuesday, start doing one of the exercises in this chapter tomorrow). You can then continue to encourage them, help them to stay on track and offer accountability for progress. Do not, however, persuade: the individual themselves needs to desire the change and it is their responsibility to do so. Solutions that the person with diabetes has not 'bought into' will not work in the long term, and may just exacerbate a feeling of failure.

Examples of reflective listening

Statement: I am feeling so down at the moment, it all feels like too much to cope with.
Reflection: You are really struggling. Life feels too demanding right now.

Statement: My diabetes is all over the place and I have my clinic appointment coming up.
Reflection: You are worried that the appointment won't go well because your diabetes hasn't been well controlled lately.

Statement: I am scared of being told off again.
Reflection: Being told off is not much fun.

Finally, make sure you have your own sources of support to lean on, so that you avoid feeling that providing support is a burden. Just as the person with depression usually needs to bring more pleasure into their lives, you do too. Follow the advice in the 'Plan more fun' section about ways to treat yourself, and do so regularly. Be aware of your own limits: if you are feeling very burdened by your role as supporter, or feel out of your depth in terms of what your loved one needs, then do get the advice of a professional. Speak to your GP or diabetes centre about an NHS referral for psychological support, or explore one of the agencies listed at the end of this chapter.

Advice for Healthcare Professionals

Diabetes clinicians play a key role in being able to identify, assist and enable support for the person with depression. The NICE Diabetes in Adults Quality Standard (National Institute for Health and Clinical Excellence, 2011) supports the diabetes National Service Framework (Department of Health, 2007) and states the need for people with diabetes to be assessed for psychological problems, which are then managed appropriately. They advise that healthcare professionals ensure they have adequate training to assess psychological problems in people with diabetes (such as depression, but also anxiety, fear of low blood sugar, eating disorders and problems coping with the diagnosis) and are familiar with referral pathways to ensure psychological problems are managed appropriately.

Simple depression screening questions for healthcare professionals

The following two questions have been demonstrated to be effective in detecting depression in routine consultations.

'During the past month, have you often been bothered by feeling down, depressed, or hopeless?'
'During the past month, have you often been bothered by feeling little interest or pleasure in doing things?'

A positive answer to either one of these questions warrants further assessment.

In the context of stretched NHS resources, adequate referral pathways are not always in place to offer the support that is needed for people with diabetes and psychological difficulties. Referrals for psychological intervention are often only possible for those patients with moderate to severe depression.

For those with mild depression, or indeed who do not want to be referred for further intervention, active monitoring is advised (National Institute for Health and Clinical Excellence, 2009). It is important for diabetes clinicians to be aware of other (non-NHS) routes of support for the person with diabetes, including resources that may be available online or informally. See the 'Further Reading' at the end of this chapter for more information.

Active monitoring

Discuss the presenting problem(s) and any concerns.
Provide information about depression.
Arrange a further assessment, normally within two weeks.
Be proactive about making contact if the patient does not attend appointments.

Healthcare professionals need also to be sensitive to cultural differences in the way emotional difficulties might be viewed by their patients. The American Psychological Society encourages practitioners, regardless of their ethnic/racial background, to be aware of how their own cultural background, experiences, attitudes, values and biases might influence psychological processes. They suggest that helping professionals might routinely ask themselves, 'Is it appropriate for me to view this client any differently than I would if they were from my own ethnic or cultural group?' (American Psychological Society, 2012). Inviting representatives from local places of worship/cultural communities to offer training in how to discuss emotional distress sensitively with members of the target population is a useful way to inform and correct any possible prejudices or stereotypes.

Clinical guidelines (National Institute for Health and Clinical Excellence, 2009) advise always asking a patient with depression and a chronic physical health problem directly about suicidal ideation and intent. If a patient presents considerable immediate risk to themselves or others, they need to be referred urgently to specialist mental health services and provided with increased support, such as more frequent clinical contact. Clinicians are sometimes wary of 'opening up a can of worms' by asking about suicidal intent, and even emotional issues more broadly, but that can of worms is there whether you are the one to open it up or not! You may feel a pressure to 'fix' the patient in emotional distress, but do not underestimate the value of your patient simply being allowed to express what they are feeling and have it heard. This in itself is very therapeutic.

How to ask about suicidal ideation

'When feeling low in the way you are describing, it is common to have thoughts that life might not be worth living, or of hurting ourselves in some way. Have you had any thoughts like this recently?'

Most importantly, do not belittle how your simple actions in a consultation can make all the difference. Asking how your patient is feeling and what is happening that is important to them, listening and then normalizing are all key strategies that can be used in the time-pressed consultation. Simply being told that what they are experiencing is normal, and that many people with diabetes struggle in similar ways, can be very therapeutic for your patients in emotional distress.

References

Ali, S., Stone, M., Peters, J., Davies, M. and Khunti, K. (2006). The prevalence of co-morbid depression in adults with Type 2 diabetes: a systematic review and meta-analysis. *Diabetic Medicine*, 23, 1165–73.

American Psychiatric Association (2000). *Diagnostic and Statistical Manual of Mental Disorders*, 4th edn, text revision (DSM-IV-TR). American Psychiatric Press, Washington, D.C.

American Psychological Society (2012). Guidelines for Providers of Psychological Services to Ethnic, Linguistic, and Culturally Diverse Populations. www.apa .org/pi/oema/resources/policy/provider-guidelines.aspx. Accessed April 2012.

Barnard, K., Lloyd, C. and Holt, R. (2012). Psychological burden of diabetes and what it means to people with diabetes. In K. Barnard and C. Lloyd (eds), *Psychology and Diabetes Care: A Practical Guide*. Springer-Verlag, London.

Barnard, K., Skinner, T. and Peveler, R. (2006). The prevalence of co-morbid depression in adults with Type 1 diabetes: systematic literature review. *Diabetic Medicine*, 23, 445–8.

Beck , Aaron (1970). *Depression: Causes and Treatment*. Philadelphia: University of Pennsylvania Press. (Originally published as *Depression: Clinical, Experimental, and Theoretical Aspects*. Harper and Row, New York, 1967.)

Blair, Linda (2008). *Straight Talking*. Piatkus, London.

Butler, Gillian and Hope, Tony (1995). *Manage Your Mind*. Oxford University Press, Oxford.

Ciechanowski, P. S., Katon, W. J. and Russon, J. E. (2000). Depression and diabetes: impact of depressive symptoms on adherence, function, and costs. *Archives of Internal Medicine*, 160, 3278–85.

Department of Health (2007). NSF Diabetes. www.dh.gov.uk/en/Publications andstatistics/Publications/PublicationsPolicyAndGuidance/Browsable /DH_4096591.

Gary, T. L., Crum, R. M., Cooper-Patrick, L., Ford, D. and Brancati, F. L. (2000). Depressive symptoms and metabolic control in African-Americans with type 2 diabetes. *Diabetes Care*, 23(1), 23–9.

Greenberger, Dennis and Padesky, Christine (1995). *Mind Over Mood*. Guilford Press, New York.

Hermanns, N., Kulzer, B., Krichbaum, M., Kubiak, T. and Haak, T. (2005) Affective and anxiety disorders in a German sample of diabetic patients: prevalence, comorbidity and risk factors. *Diabetic Medicine*, 22(3), 293–300.

Hermanns, N. Kulzer, B., Krichbaum, M., Kubiak, T. and Haak, T. (2006). How to screen for depression and emotional problem in patients with diabetes: comparison of screening characteristics of depression questionnaires, measurement of diabetes-specific emotional problems and standard clinical assessment. *Diabetologia*, 49(3) 469–77.

Ismail, K. (2010). Unraveling the pathogenesis of the depression–diabetes link. In W. Katon, M. Mario and N. Sartorius (eds), *Depression and Diabetes*. Wiley-Blackwell, Chichester.

Kroenke, K., Spitzer, R. L. and Williams, J. B. (2001). The PHQ-9: validity of a brief depression severity measure. *Journal of General Internal Medicine*, 16(9), 606–13.

Mezuk, B., Eaton, W. W., Albrecht, S. and Golden, S. H. (2008). Depression and type 2 diabetes over the lifespan: a meta-analysis. *Diabetes Care*, 31(12), 2383–90.

National Institute for Health and Clinical Excellence (2009). Depression in adults with a chronic physical health problem: treatment and management. http://publications.nice.org.uk/depression-in-adults-with-a-chronic-physical-health-problem-cg91. CG91. Accessed 22 November 2012.

National Institute for Health and Clinical Excellence (2011). Diabetes in adults quality standard. QS6. http://publications.nice.org.uk/diabetes-in-adults-quality-standard-qs6. Accessed 8 December 2012.

Polonsky, W., Anderson, B., Lohrer, P., Welch, G., Jacobson, A., Aponte, J. and Schwartz, C. (1995). Assessment of diabetes-related distress. *Diabetes Care*, 18, 754–60.

Polonsky, William (1999). *Diabetes Burnout*. American Diabetes Association, Alexandria, VA.

Pouwer, F., Beekman, T. F. and Nijpels, G. (2003) Rates and risks for co-morbid depression in patients with Type 2 diabetes mellitus: results from a community-based study. *Diabetologia*, 46(7), 892–8.

Pouwer, F., Geelhoed-Duijveestihn, H. L. M., Tack, C. J., Bazelmans, E., Beekman, A.-J., Heine, R. J. and Snoek, F. J. (2010). Prevalence of comorbid depression is high in out-patients with Type 1 or Type 2 diabetes mellitus: results from the three out-patient clinics in the Netherlands. *Diabetic Medicine* 27, 217–24.

Pouwer, F. and Hermanns, N. (2009). Insulin therapy and quality of life: a review. *Diabetes/Metabolism Research and Reviews*, 25 (suppl. 1), S4–S10.

Rowe, Dorothy (2003). *Depression: The Way Out of Your Prison*, 3rd edn. Routledge, London.

Rubin, R. (2000). Diabetes and quality of life. *Diabetes Spectrum*, 13, 21.

Willis, T. (1674). *Pharmaceutice Rationalis: Sive Diatriba De Medicamentorum Operationibus in Humano Corpore*. E Theatro Sheldoniano, Oxford.

World Health Organization (2012). Depression. www.who.int/mental_health/management/depression/definition/en/. Accessed April 2012.

Further Reading and Resources

K. Barnard and C. Lloyd (eds) (2012). *Psychology and Diabetes Care: A Practical Guide*. Springer-Verlag, London.
Linda Blair (2008). *Straight Talking*. Piatkus, London.
David Burns (1999). *The Feeling Good Handbook*. Random House, New York.
Gillian Butler and Tony Hope (1995). *Manage Your Mind*. Oxford University Press, Oxford.
Dennis Greenberger and Christine Padesky (1995). *Mind Over Mood*. Guilford Press, New York.
William Polonsky (1999). *Diabetes Burnout*. American Diabetes Association, Alexandria, VA.
Dorothy Rowe (2003). *Depression: The Way Out of Your Prison*, 3rd edn. Routledge, London.

Directories to Find a Therapist

British Psychological Society: www.bps.org.uk/bpslegacy/dcp.
British Association for Counselling and Psychotherapy: www.bacp.co.uk.
Positive Diabetes: www.PositiveDiabetes.com.

Useful Websites

NHS Direct: www.nhsdirect.nhs.uk.
MIND: www.mind.org.uk.
BBC Health homepage: www.bbc.co.uk/health/.
Diabetes UK: www.diabetes.org.uk.
Diabetes Research and Wellness Foundation: www.drwf.org.uk.
Positive Diabetes: www.PositiveDiabetes.com.
Diabetes forums: www.diabetes.co.uk, www.DiabetesDaily.com, www.dlife.com, www.DiabetesSisters.com.

5

Managing Fear, Anxiety and Worry

Fear. Panic. Phobia. Worry. Nervousness. All names for one of the most distressing of the human emotions – anxiety. This chapter will outline the causes of fear and anxiety and the specific ways it can affect individuals with diabetes, in particular, fear of long-term complications, anxiety about hypoglycaemia, fear of needles/blood glucose testing and general worry. Strategies to tackle and overcome anxiety will be outlined.

What Causes Anxiety?

Anxiety is a natural response that has evolved in us as a reaction to situations that we perceive as dangerous. In our evolutionary history, our ancestors needed fast and effective responses to survive in a hostile world, in which predators were many and often unpredictable. Three reactions to anxiety were established within us: the fight, flight and freeze responses.

Some dangers, such as facing up to a predator, required a fight response. Plenty of oxygen and tense muscles were needed. Other risks involved fleeing. To run from an animal our ancestors required an accelerated heart rate to ensure plenty of oxygen was reaching their cells. For other threats it was appropriate to freeze. Perhaps the predator had not seen the individual yet, and if he stayed very still the animal would not notice him. This would require very rigid muscles and shallow breath, to prevent breathing from being visible.

These responses were hugely effective in the environment in which they evolved. Those humans who had the most effective fight/flight/flee

Diabetes and Wellbeing: Managing the Psychological and Emotional Challenges of Diabetes Types 1 and 2, First Edition. Dr Jen Nash.
© 2013 John Wiley & Sons, Ltd. Published 2013 by John Wiley & Sons, Ltd.

response were the ones who survived to pass their genes on to subsequent generations. The problem is that against the 'dangers' that are present in our modern-day lives – dealing with your specific fears about diabetes, the meeting with your boss, giving a speech at your wedding or the flight abroad on holiday – this strong physiological anxiety reaction is not so helpful. Our biological responses have not evolved to adapt to our modern-day environments, in which anxiety is generally a reaction to important events we find challenging or upsetting, such as:

Illness
The death of a loved one
Being in an accident
Redundancy or job loss
Job promotion
Giving a speech in public
A new life stage such as parenthood, or the children leaving home
Learning from others that is significant for our survival, e.g. snakes will bite you, a sensation in your chest is a heart attack
Observations that may induce fear (reading an article in the newspaper about a plane crash)
Believing you are rejected, embarrassed, humiliated or put down.

Are You Currently Struggling with Anxiety?

Changes caused by anxiety (Butler and Hope, 1995)

Physical reactions

Racing heart
Sweaty palms
Muscle tension
Flushed cheeks
Light-headedness

Thoughts

Worries and catastrophic thoughts
Overestimating danger
Underestimating your ability to cope
Underestimating the help available

Moods and emotions

Anxious
Panicky
Nervous
Irritable

Behaviours

Trying to control events to prevent danger
Avoiding situations where anxiety might occur
Leaving situations when anxiety begins to occur
Aiming for perfection to control events

You may well recognize some of the signs of anxiety in these lists, as the presence of these feelings, thoughts and moods to some degree are a normal aspect of life. Perhaps you are not currently experiencing any or many anxiety symptoms at all, in which case you can move ahead to another chapter, or read the information that follows as a reference in case your situation may change in the future. Or maybe you are at the other extreme, and you are struggling with significant anxiety currently. Wherever you are, the following sections will help you to understand why you are feeling this way and how to start right away to gain control over your mood.

Specific Fears that Affect People with Diabetes

Three common anxieties that affect those with diabetes are:

Fear of hypoglycaemia
Fear of long-term complications
Fear of needles/blood glucose monitoring

Each of these will be addressed independently. At the end of the chapter, coping with more generalized types of anxiety and worries will be covered.

Fear of hypoglycaemia

First, let us remind ourselves what hypoglycaemia (sometimes called a 'hypo' for short) is. In diabetes, the body can't regulate blood glucose levels properly. This means that food intake, medication and activity levels need to be closely monitored to ensure that the levels of glucose required for good health remain stable. Hypoglycaemia is the medical term for the occasions when blood glucose level falls too low. When blood glucose levels are low, a series of physical reactions take place. These include:

feeling weak
feeling light-headed
feeling shaky
feeling confused
sweating
hunger
tiredness
blurred vision
pins and needles around your mouth
finding it hard to concentrate
headaches
feeling tearful
increased heart rate
becoming stroppy or stubborn.

Hypoglycaemia can occur in individuals with type 1 or type 2 diabetes, although it occurs more often in those with type 1 because of the delicate balance that needs to be maintained between food and insulin requirements and energy expended.

A hypo is most likely to occur when:

you have missed a meal or snack
you have had too much insulin
your meal was delayed
you did not have enough carbohydrate (such as pasta, rice, bread, cereal or
    potatoes) at your last meal
you did some strenuous exercise without taking extra carbohydrate or
    reducing your insulin dose to allow for it
you have got too hot (a hot bath or being in the sun for too long increases
    the rate at which insulin is absorbed)
you've had too much alcohol to drink.

Hypoglycaemia is a frequent occurrence among many people with diabetes; mild to moderate episodes (those that you can treat on your own) occur about twice a week on average for the person with type 1. Many people with diabetes worry a lot about the possibility of a hypoglycaemic episode: in one study 25 per cent of people with diabetes reported that worrying about hypoglycaemia is a serious problem for them (Polonsky, 1999).

So why do people worry about hypoglycaemia, particularly when, in most cases, it can be treated with relative speed and ease by consuming a sugary drink or snack? Well, easy as it can be to treat, the effects of a hypo can be frightening, embarrassing, uncomfortable, unpleasant or, in their worst cases, fatal. Getting sweaty, having slurred speech, shaking uncontrollably or being confused may not seem too bad in the whole scheme of things, but having them occur in a job interview or important work meeting, whilst driving home at night or on a romantic date may not be so pleasant!

Remember that anxiety and phobias have evolutionary value. We are hard-wired to engage in actions that ensure our survival, and 'survival' can be defined broadly: we want to avoid things that will lead to possible rejection or isolation from others, and acting oddly whilst in the midst of a hypo is one example of such things. Hypos *can* be dangerous, but ordinarily people can put their potential fear into perspective and not let it change or alter their behaviour too much.

However, for some individuals, having just one aversive or frightening episode of hypoglycaemia can lead to increased anxiety about it happening again. This can lead to other behaviours, which in turn may lead to further difficulties with managing diabetes:

Running blood glucose levels higher than usual to avoid hypoglycaemia
Eating more than is needed in an attempt to keep blood glucose level elevated
Restricting activities where a hypoglycaemic episode would be more challenging to deal with, such as driving, exercising, or travelling on public transport.

In addition to having had a particularly bad experience of hypoglycaemia, three further factors may contribute to excessive worry.

A weakened ability to feel the warning signs of hypoglycaemia   The warning signs of hypoglycaemia, such as sweating and shaking, are caused by the release of the body's stress-related hormone, adrenaline. However, for some people with diabetes, their warning signs are less obvious, and so by the time they do notice the problem their blood glucose level has dropped so low that taking reparative action becomes even harder.

Inability to distinguish the feelings of hypoglycaemia from the feelings of fear
Many symptoms of hypoglycaemia, such as sweatiness or an increased heart rate, are the same as signs you would experience if you were fearful. This may lead to a spiral of confusion:

You notice your heart beating a little faster
You think, 'This could be hypoglycaemia'
This makes you nervous, so your heart beats even faster
You may think, 'Oh no, this is a symptom of hypoglycaemia ....'
You feel even more nervous and reach for the glucose to raise your blood sugar levels.

when what you really were experiencing was straightforward anxiety.

You may find predicting or estimating your blood glucose level challenging
Everyone's experience of hypoglycaemia is different; therefore, although you have probably been taught to be alert for certain signs of hypoglycaemia, your own response may be quite unique – a particular taste in your mouth or an unusual feeling in your legs.

Five strategies for overcoming your difficulties with hypoglycaemia

1. Talk to your healthcare team   If you frequently experience low blood glucose levels, the first thing that you may need is a change to your diabetes regime: your medication type, the dosage, or the timing of medication and/or food and/or activity. Your doctor and nurse will be able to help with this. If you are experiencing fewer warning signs than previously, there are ways of recovering these, through avoiding all hypos for as little as a few weeks. This needs careful planning to avoid the opposite problem of overly high blood glucose levels, but is very possible with guidance from your health professionals.

2. Immediately before checking your blood glucose, guess what the number will be   Increase your confidence in your hypo awareness by estimating what yours is before you actually test. Write down your guess in Table 5.2, then

Table 5.1   Example record of blood glucose estimates

Date/time	Estimate	Why is this your Estimate?	Actual Result
Monday 4.30 pm	3.1	My heart's beating fast	6.2

test and write down the actual result. See Table 5.1 for an example diary. If you often guess incorrectly, use the strategies that follow to help you.

Learn your unique warning signs of hypos   Everyone has their own individual 'alarm bells' (Polonsky, 1999), which are your body's way of telling you that your blood glucose is low. Keep track of what you notice going on for you when you have a hypo (obviously best thought about *after* you have recovered from one!). Is it a physical symptom (heart racing, tingling in a certain part of your body, sweating, shaking, heart palpitations) or a change in your mood or in your ability to think clearly? Using Table 5.3 as a guide, make a note of this in Table 5.4, or note it in your diary, notebook or phone, and notice if you start to see a pattern emerging.

4. Find out what works best for treating your hypoglycaemia   Experiment! Some people like to use sweet food that they might not normally indulge in, such as chocolate, but because of the high fat content, chocolate can actually be slow to raise blood glucose levels sufficiently. Simple sugars contained in orange juice, glucose tablets, energy drinks, sweets and honey can act more quickly. It is very frustrating to eat a snack and for it not to work effectively, so try a variety of foods and see what works for you. Once you have found what works best, try to always carry some of it with you.

5. If you tend to think you are having a hypo reaction even when you are not, try a breathing exercise   If you realize that you are often mistaking anxiety for hypoglycaemia, a quick relaxation exercise can help control your reaction, giving you a minute to discover whether or not you are experiencing hypoglycaemia. Try the following quick exercise:

Sit comfortably in a chair
Close your eyes
Take a slow, deep breath in through your nose so your lungs are full
Hold this breath for the count of 3 seconds

Table 5.2   Record of blood glucose estimates

Date/time	Estimate	Why is this your Estimate?	Actual Result

Table 5.3   Example blood glucose alarm bells diary

Day	My Alarm Bells
Monday	Couldn't concentrate on my work Felt hot Noticed my palms were sweaty
Tuesday	Felt hot Snapped at my sister Sweaty

Table 5.4   Blood glucose alarm bells diary

Day	My Alarm Bells
Monday	
Tuesday	
Wednesday	
Thursday	
Friday	
Saturday	
Sunday	

Breathe out through your mouth as fully as possible for a count of 5 seconds

Repeat this sequence for two more breaths

Open your eyes and notice any subtle differences in how you feel, both in your body and your mind

With a bit of practice, over time you will be able to notice a feeling of relaxation that comes with this breathing exercise.

Once you feel comfortable with the technique, begin to practise it when you are having symptoms that you are not sure are hypoglycaemic. If they weaken it is likely to be a false alarm, but in the beginning *always* test your blood glucose level to see if you are correct. With frequent practice, over time you can expect the false alarms to occur less frequently.

Using CBT to Manage Fear of Hypoglycaemia

Case study: Alicia

Alicia has had diabetes for many years. Recently she been finding it difficult to figure out if she is having a hypo or not. If in doubt she tends to eat a snack to avoid getting into any embarrassing situations.

Step 1: What is the situation or event?

Noticing physical symptoms that I think may be the sign of a hypo

Thinking that I may be hypoglycaemic

Step 2: What do you tell yourself? What are the thoughts you notice running through your mind?

'Do I have low blood sugar right now?'

'I'm pretty sure I'm low.'

'I'm not sure if this is a hypo or not. If it is and I don't act on it I'm going to make a fool of myself/collapse/get into a difficult situation.'

'I hate not knowing.'

'I feel so stupid. Other people with diabetes don't have this problem.'

Step 3: What is happening in your body and what do you do?

Mood – fearful, anxious, scared, embarrassed

Body sensations – heart beating fast, shallow breathing

Behaviours – stop what I'm doing and look for something to eat

Step 4: Challenge your thoughts by asking yourself some helpful questions

What is the evidence for and against this thought?

Is thinking this way helping me?

Are there other ways of thinking about this situation?

If a friend told me they were thinking this way, how would I respond?

Am I thinking in 'all or nothing' terms?

What other points of view are there?

How would someone else think about this?

How else could I think about it?

How would I think about this if I were feeling better?

What are the facts of the case?

How can I find out which way of thinking fits the facts best?

What is the evidence?

Could I be making a mistake in the way I am thinking?

Am I thinking straight?

Am I pressurizing myself?

Am I using the language of the extremist?

What is the worst thing that could happen?

Step 5: Come up with an alternative, balanced thought

'Do I have low blood sugar right now?' I am going to follow my plan: guess what my blood glucose level is and then test and make a note of the actual figure.

'I'm pretty sure I'm low.' I'm learning how to figure out the difference between *actual* hypoglycaemia and *fear* of hypoglycaemia.

'I'm not sure if this is a hypo or not. If it is and I don't act on it I'm going to make a fool of myself/collapse/get into a difficult situation.' If my blood glucose level is low, I will eat/drink [insert your best food/drink for combating hypos].

'I hate not knowing.' Although I feel low, I am just anxious. Although I do not like feeling this way, it will pass. Every time I can be aware of the anxiety, I am getting better.

'I feel so stupid. Other people with diabetes don't have this problem.' Everyone with diabetes struggles with some aspect of it at some point. This is my struggle, but it will not be around for ever, I'm on my way to recovery.

Dealing with the Fear of Long-Term Complications

Many people with diabetes are apprehensive of all the new demands that accompany the diagnosis. There is a lot to adjust to in a short time: the uncertainty of the balance between medication, food and activity, and ever present thoughts of 'What if I get it wrong?' looming in the background. Implementing new health regimes, starting new behaviours and routines, ending old ones . . . these are just the *daily* challenges of living with diabetes. The possibility of future challenges in the form of long-term complications can also be a very powerful fear.

Fear of long-term complications can be one of the most undermining to good health, but also the least often voiced and understood. Developing problems in the long term can be so intangible – some individuals are fortunate enough to develop no long-term complications at all, whilst others are hugely affected by them. There can also be a sense of injustice with long-term complications: some people who manage their blood glucose levels consistently well still go on to develop complications, while those who fail to take care of their health are fortunate enough to avoid them. Confusing and unfair, right?

So what are long-term complications? They can include:

kidney disease (nephropathy)
eye disease
cataracts
glaucoma
retinopathy
nerve disease (neuropathy)
heart disease
peripheral arterial disease
cerebrovascular disease
diabetic foot disease
skin disease

But what can you actually do about the daily worry? Here are some strategies for dealing with the fear of long-term complications.

Keep your thoughts about diabetes risks in perspective

Yes, people with diabetes *do* develop long-term complications, some for no good reason, and this is, like many aspects of health, unfair. However, newer, more refined medicines for both type 1 and type 2 are being developed all the time, along with more advanced technologies for dealing with it: continuous blood glucose monitors, insulin pumps, at-home blood pressure monitors, and still more to come. The future is brighter for all of us (both with and without diabetes) as the medical field advances. Did you know that one of the first insulin treatment 'guinea pigs' in 1922 – Elizabeth Evans Hughes – lived well into her seventies? Read all about her in Box 5.1. Just think how far insulin has advanced since then.

Box 5.1 The insulin guinea pig (Polonsky, 1999)

Two scientists named Banting and Best discovered insulin in the early 1920s in their laboratory in Canada. One of their first patients was a 15-year-old girl called Elizabeth Evans Hughes. In the early twentieth century people with a diagnosis of diabetes faced an early death, and Elizabeth was very underweight and frail when this newly discovered hormone was offered to her. She started taking two insulin injections a day under Dr Banting's care, began to recover quickly and returned home, staying in regular touch with him by letter until 1926. Nothing was heard from Elizabeth after this point, and it was assumed she had died. After all, the early insulins were impure and she was without the benefit of the blood glucose-monitoring technology we have now to adjust doses as necessary. In 1980, a historian named Professor Michael Bliss was interested to research her fate and the complications she had suffered before her inevitable early death. To his surprise and excitement, he tracked down a 73-year-old Elizabeth still alive and in good health, with minimal complications caused by diabetes. At a time when children with type 1 diabetes rarely survived more than three decades, this can be viewed as a miracle of hope for those fearful of long-term complications today.

Indeed, there are health risks with diabetes, but there are risks you take with your health every day. Not sure you believe me? Have you ever been in a car on a busy road? Taken a flight? Set a Christmas pudding alight? These are behaviours with the chance of a negative outcome, yet we engage in them because we decide that the risk is worth the benefit of engaging in them. The risk of getting hurt while travelling may be low, but then people are in road traffic accidents every day. So yes, there are risks with diabetes, but living a full life also includes elements of risk taking, so do your best to keep these in perspective. See the next section for specific CBT strategies to help you with this.

Remind yourself of the actual facts

For some, the identification of the first sign of long-term complications leads to a feeling of catastrophe. If you have been diagnosed with such a complication you may feel very pessimistic and certain that you are now on a downward course of ill health. However, in many cases the opposite is true: the diagnosis of a particular complication of diabetes can bring a fresh motivation to care well for one's health, especially given that changes to health behaviour can halt if not reverse some complications. Many people cite this as the time when they began to be more proactive about caring for their diabetes health. Remind yourself of this, perhaps with a supportive statement written in your diary or on your computer screensaver where you will notice it often: 'Every time I make a wise health choice I am moving further away from developing complications.'

Focus on what you can control: diabetes self-care

One of the most effective health-increasing tools you have at your disposal is a feeling of self-control. This is because it puts you in a position of power – feeling that you *can* make changes that will lead to better health outcomes. These changes might be exercising more, making a healthier food swap, testing your blood glucose once more per day than you currently do, making that healthcare appointment you've been putting off for ages. Although a low level of anxiety about developing complications can be helpful, in that it can keep you motivated, knowing that you can take positive action, and that your actions do matter, is an incredibly good antidote to fear. Use the information and support available in this book, and in other resources you have access to, to help you focus on what *is* controllable, and your fears about the long-term effects of diabetes will diminish.

Using CBT to Manage the Fear of Long-Term Complications

Case study: Henry

Henry has had diabetes for a number of years now and at his most recent review he was diagnosed with neuropathy. He had avoided thinking about developing long-term complications and had simply hoped that they would not affect him. He was scared about what this meant.

Step 1: What is the situation or event?

Feeling the symptoms of the tingling in my legs and remembering the conversation when the doctor told me the news

Step 2: What do you tell yourself? What are the thoughts you notice running through your mind?

'I'm scared.'
'What does this mean for my future?'
'I'm going to get really unwell.'
'This is the beginning of a downward spiral of ill health.'

Step 3: What is happening in your body and what do you do?

Mood – fearful, anxious, scared
Body sensations – heart beating fast, shallow breathing
Behaviours – keeping busy, wanting to distract myself by having a
    cigarette

Step 4: Challenge your thoughts by asking yourself some helpful questions

What is the evidence for and against this thought?
Is thinking this way helping me?
Are there other ways of thinking about this situation?
If a friend told me they were thinking this way, how would I respond?
Am I thinking in 'all or nothing' terms?
What other points of view are there?

How would someone else think about this?
How else could I think about it?
How would I think about this if I were feeling better?
What are the facts of the case?
How can I find out which way of thinking fits the facts best?
What is the evidence?
Could I be making a mistake in the way I am thinking?
Am I thinking straight?
Am I pressurizing myself?
Am I using the language of the extremist?
What is the worst thing that could happen?

Step 5: Come up with an alternative, balanced thought

'I'm scared.' The thought of long-term complications *is* scary. But so is the thought of being in a car accident and I still travel on the roads! I am going to try and keep this in perspective.

'What does this mean for my future?' I cannot control whether I eventually do develop more long-term problems, but what I can control is how I care for my diabetes health today.

'I'm going to get really unwell.' I can choose to be somewhat grateful that this complication has been diagnosed. It means it can be monitored and prevented from getting worse than it would have done undetected.

'This is the beginning of a downward spiral of ill health.' I am going to choose to create an upward spiral of good health, by cutting down one cigarette a day this week/going for a 10-minute walk every other day.

Needle phobia

For many people with diabetes, injections and blood glucose testing are simply a necessary part of life. But for many, both the newly diagnosed and those who have been managing the condition for longer, the injection and blood glucose-testing process can be very distressing. But what turns a plain dislike of needles into an actual phobia? Well, a phobia is an extreme or irrational fear or aversion to something. Along with needle phobia, fear of public speaking, fear of the dentist and fear of heights are some very common phobias encountered among the general population.

A small degree of dislike of needles is perfectly normal – most people would avoid them if they possibly could. But this fear is greatly heightened in people with needle phobia, to the point where they cannot bear the thought of injections. Needle phobia is common in the general population. Some studies suggest the rate of occurrence is at least 10 per cent (Hamilton, 1995), although it is likely that the actual number is larger, as many sufferers simply avoid all medical treatment.

The symptoms of needle phobia vary greatly from one individual to another. The main feature is anxiety at the thought of injections or blood glucose testing. This may be associated with feeling dizzy and light-headed, a dry mouth, palpitations, sweating, trembling, over-breathing, feeling sick and even fainting, and lead to attempts to avoid them.

Why does it occur?   Although it can be difficult to be entirely sure what causes a phobia of needles, the most common causes are thought to be:

1. An upsetting experience of needles when young, for example, a painful procedure at the hospital or at the dentist
2. A fear that has been 'modelled' by an adult close to the child, either through actual observation of their fear, or being told a story that implied injections and needles were very painful.
3. There is also evolutionary value to a fear of needles. In the past, an individual who feared being gored by a horn or stabbed with a knife was less likely to die in accidents or in encounters with hostile animals or other humans. Before the twentieth century, even an otherwise non-fatal puncture wound had a reasonable chance of causing a fatal infection. So a trait that had positive survival value in our evolutionary history now has the opposite effect, as it means people struggle to engage in using the needle that will save their life.

Needle phobia and diabetes   Mollema, Snoek, Pouwer et al. (2000) investigated individuals with type 1 diabetes and a fear of self-injecting or of self-testing. They found that high levels of fear were associated not just with poorer adherence to the diabetes treatment regimen, but with more diabetes-related distress overall and poorer general wellbeing.

How to overcome needle phobia   Gaining skills of relaxation and confidence is the key to making injections less painful and less anxiety-provoking. You will develop confidence over time and with practice, using a combination of relaxation and developing your own personal 'fear hierarchy'. A fear hierarchy is a series of steps that you could take to overcome your fear, from the least feared to the most feared. A special note if your fear is such that you feel faint, or do faint: fainting is associated with a sudden drop in blood pressure, which can be prevented by tensing up your muscles instead of attempting to relax, so use the 'applied tension' technique, described below.

Applied tension to prevent fainting   Tighten the muscle groups in your arms, legs and torso all at once and hold this position for about 5 seconds. Let go of the tension momentarily and then tense up again. Practise this while sitting down at home somewhere quiet twice a day, starting with a few minutes and building up to 10 minutes. Once you are comfortable doing this sitting down, progress to a standing position. Once this is familiar, start to tackle your fear hierarchy using applied tension as you work through the steps.

Create your own fear hierarchy   A fear hierarchy is a series of actions to take in order to overcome your fear. Using Table 5.5 as a guide, make a list in Table 5.6 of the actions that you are now avoiding in relation to injecting or blood glucose testing. Put them in order of difficulty, beginning with the least feared action and progressing to the most feared. The first could be something you find relatively easy, e.g. looking at the insulin pen, holding it in your hand, or perhaps watching someone else inject.

As you can see, the first step should be one that may be frightening, but in a way that is much more manageable than the final steps. Like a ladder, you need to take one step at a time to reach the top of it. It is impossible to leap from the first to the final step in one go and you do not need to. Just focus on the next step. Once you have identified the 'rungs' on your ladder you can start to climb it. Follow the instructions below for each step, starting with step 1.

1. Rate the level of fear you have in relation to the step, on a scale of 0–10, where 0 is no fear at all and 10 is the most fear you could possibly experience. Do not spend too long deciding upon the number (e.g. am I a 6 or a 7?). It is usually advisable to go with the first number that occurs to you.
2. Using Table 5.7 as a guide, make a note of your 'Start' rating in Table 5.8.
3. As you engage in the feared activity, use the relaxation exercise described below.

Table 5.5 Example fear hierarchy to tackle needle phobia

Step	Situation
1	Look at pictures and photos of insulin and injection pens
2	Talk to people about injecting
3	Look at my insulin pen
4	Hold the insulin pen in my hand
5	Watch someone else inject
6	Draw up the correct insulin dose and prepare to inject
7	Hold the pen above my skin and imagine I am injecting
8	Hold the pen so the needle touches my skin
9	Hold the pen so the needle touches my skin and imagine I am pushing it into my flesh
10	Inject (perhaps into the stomach first: many people find it less painful as there are few nerve endings there)
11	Inject in other parts of body: thigh, buttock, etc.
12	Inject in different geographical locations: at a friend's house, in a restaurant, on a train

Relaxation exercise

Sit comfortably in a chair
Close your eyes
Take a slow, deep breath in so your lungs are full
Hold this breath for the count of 3 seconds
Breathe out as fully as possible for a count of 5 seconds
Repeat this sequence for two more breaths
Open your eyes and notice any subtle differences in how you feel, both in your body and in your mind

Table 5.6 Fear hierarchy to tackle needle phobia

Step	Situation
1	
2	
3	
4	
5	
6	
7	
8	
9	
10	
11	
12	

With a bit of practice, over time you will be able to notice a feeling of relaxation

Once you feel comfortable with the technique, begin to practise it with your eyes open when you are working through your fear hierarchy

4. Stay in each scenario until the anxiety starts to subside and you begin to feel better. Anxiety cannot continue at heightened levels indefinitely. Keep checking in with yourself and rating your anxiety level from 0

Table 5.7   Example record of overcoming fear

Day	Step Tackled	Fear Rating at Start (0–10)	Fear Rating Mid-way (0–10)	Fear Rating at End (0–10)	What I Learned
Mon	1	6	3	2	My fear did decrease! This step was pretty easy.
Tues	1	4	2	1	I can move on to step 2 now.
Wed	2	8	7	6	Much more scared this time. But I stayed with the fear and it went down.
Thurs	2	8	5	5	I'm pleased that the fear is decreasing, although not as quickly as I would like.
Fri					
Sat					
Sun					

to 10. When you notice it has decreased by one point on the scale, encourage yourself by mentally saying 'well done!'

5. Continue at each step and practise on a number of different occasions until you can do it with a fear level of 3 or below. Then move on to the next step on your fear hierarchy.

6. Practise every day if possible, or as often as you can, in order to maintain momentum and prevent avoidance behaviour. You might want to plan a time into your routine when you will be free to practise each day, for example after breakfast or after work.

Table 5.8 Record of overcoming fear

Day	Step Tackled	Fear Rating at Start (0–10)	Fear Rating Mid-way (0–10)	Fear Rating at End (0–10)	What I Learned
Mon					
Tues					
Wed					
Thurs					
Fri					
Sat					
Sun					

7. Plan a treat for yourself as a reward after you have practised (see Chapter 8 for ideas on rewards).
8. Take your time and progress at a pace that suits you. There is no rush. You probably developed this fear over time, so it will take time to recover from it. It does not matter how slowly you go. Just as a child falls over many times when he or she is learning to walk, there will be times when

you feel a bit set back. This is a normal part of change and progress. On the days when you are struggling, go easy on yourself.

9. If you get stuck at a particular step and are fearful to move on, think about how you could make the next step easier. Is there a time of day when you are less tired or feel more resilient to do things that are outside your comfort zone? Or could talking to a loved one and having them sit with you while you practise be helpful?

Using CBT to Manage your Fear of Needles

Case study: Donna

Donna had always disliked injections and hated having to get travel vaccinations when she went travelling a few years ago. Recently diagnosed, she was finding it difficult to come to terms with the fact that she would need to inject herself every day for the rest of her life. If she could get away with it, she was beginning to avoid both injecting and testing her blood glucose as often as she should.

Step 1: What is the situation or event?

Thinking about injecting
Knowing I have to inject
Seeing my injection pen/equipment
Someone asking me, 'Do you need to have your insulin?'

Step 2: What do you tell yourself? What are the thoughts you notice running through your mind?

'I hate all these needles.'
'I just want to be normal.'
'I feel like a pincushion!'
'Other people will see me inject and think I'm a drug user.'

Step 3: What is happening in your body and what do you do?

Mood – fearful, anxious
Body sensations – heart beating fast, shallow breathing
Behaviours – avoid injecting, pretend to go to another room to inject so no one will say anything

Step 4: Challenge your thoughts by asking yourself some helpful questions

What is the evidence for and against this thought?
Is thinking this way helping me?
Are there other ways of thinking about this situation?
If a friend told me they were thinking this way, how would I respond?
Am I thinking in 'all or nothing' terms?
What other points of view are there?
How would someone else think about this?
How else could I think about it?
How would I think about this if I were feeling better?
What are the facts of the case?
How can I find out which way of thinking fits the facts best?
What is the evidence?
Could I be making a mistake in the way I am thinking?
Am I thinking straight?
Am I pressurizing myself?
Am I using the language of the extremist?
What is the worst thing that could happen?

Step 5: Come up with an alternative, balanced thought

'I hate all these needles.' I do not like the needles but I can recover.
'I just want to be normal.' I am normal. I am learning how to get over
    this by following my plan. I just need to focus on the stage I am on.
    Every time I can be aware of the anxiety, I am getting better.
'I feel like a pincushion!' Having these injections is keeping me alive.
    After I've injected or tested my blood I will do something nice for
    myself: have a cup of tea, watch TV, read my book or phone a
    friend.
'Other people will see me inject and think I'm a drug user.' Drug users
    do not tend to do it publicly like I do! If someone is looking they are
    just curious, not necessarily judging. I too look at unusual things,
    like someone with a plaster cast or multi-coloured hair.
'I hate the feeling of injecting.' Although I do not like feeling this way,
    I am not in danger. There is a difference between pain and danger.
    Pain may not be pleasant, but my life is not at risk.

Overcoming General Anxieties and Worries

A certain amount of everyday worry is normal for everyone, and indeed worry does have necessary and positive survival attributes. It can prompt you to take precautions (e.g. fastening your seat belt or buying insurance) or avoid risky behaviours (e.g. angering dangerous animals, or driving after drinking alcohol). Worry has therefore evolved as a way to help us solve problems and keep ourselves safe from harm. If our ancestors had not worried about how secure from danger their cave was, they would not have survived long! The problem is that many of the worries in our modern day lives are not so practically solvable. Worries can eat away at our sense of wellbeing and it can feel like we have no control over them.

Some of the ways worry can affect you (Butler and Hope, 1995)

How worry affects your thinking: what is on your mind

Interferes with concentration and with your ability to give something your full attention
Focuses your attention onto yourself and your own concerns
Makes it hard to make decisions
Increases your ability to notice negative things and to concentrate on these more than other things (selective attention)
Makes you more pessimistic, so you tend to predict the worst
Makes you problem-focused, so your mind leaps from one worry to the next.

How worry affects your behaviour: the things you do

Makes you less efficient (either over-careful, or unwittingly careless)
Interferes with your performance
Makes you rely more on others and less on yourself
Leads you to do things less confidently

How worry affects your feelings: your emotions

Makes you feel muddled or confused
Makes you feel apprehensive and fearful
Makes you feel out of control
Makes you feel overwhelmed or that you can't cope

How worry affects your body

Reduces your ability to relax and to sleep well
Makes you weary and tired
Makes you tense
Gives you headaches

Have a 'worry time'

Compartmentalizing worry is helpful. Set yourself a 'worry time' when your only job is to worry intentionally. Decide upon a time during the day when you will be free to have some uninterrupted time on your own. Perhaps it is first thing in the morning, or when you get home from work. Choose a time you can commit to and set an alarm on your phone to remind you. The duration of your worry time is up to you; I suggest starting with 30 minutes (often people are pleasantly surprised that they have run out of things to worry about after 10 minutes!).

When it is your worry time, sit in a quiet place where you will not be interrupted. Set a timer for 30 minutes. Have a pad and paper and start writing down your worries. Do not think too hard at this stage – just let them all spill out onto the page. Once the stream has slowed, put your pen down and read your worries back. Give each worry a rating of 1, 2 or 3:

1 = a worry you can definitely do something about
2 = a worry you may be able to do something about
3 = a worry you cannot do anything about

Now, tackle the worries you have marked with a 1. Problem-solve: what are the actions you could take or conversations you could have to tackle these? Put a time/date by when you are going to commit to doing each action you need to take.

Now move on to the worries you have marked with a 2. If you could not fail, what would you do? All ideas are good ideas at this point so do not censor your thoughts. Scribble down your ideas and see if any of them are feasible. If so, again put a time/date by when you are going to commit to doing each action you need to take.

Finally, examine the number 3s. Again, brainstorm and see if there might be some ideas you can generate for tackling this worry. If not, that is OK. Some worries cannot be immediately solved. However, by using this process you will see that there is a beginning and an end to your worries; they are not as endless as they seem when they are running around inside your head.

Once your timer has gone off, or you have reached the end of your worries, put your pad away until the same time tomorrow. Of course, your brain will continue to try and draw you back to your worries, so just notice them and respond internally, 'Oh look, I'm worrying again. I have dealt with the worries today and Worry Time is now not until 6 pm tomorrow. So right now I am going to choose to distract myself.'

Distraction

Distraction is helpful as it allows you to shift your focus from the physical sensations or thoughts that are likely to be fuelling your anxiety. As you know by now, your thoughts are central to your experience, so by getting absorbed in something else you can distance yourself from the source of the worry. Decide in advance on a few different ways of distracting yourself.

Distraction outside the home

Count the number of red/blue cars you see
Count the shops or objects beginning with the letter 'T', or another letter
Count the number of dog walkers you pass
Focus on something in great detail: a plant, or the chair you are sitting on.
   Mentally describe the colour, shades and textures
Mentally visit a 'happy place' (a memory of a nice time in your past)

Distraction at home

Organize a drawer
Write a shopping list
Read a book
Text a friend
Fix or mend something
Paint your nails

See Chapter 4 for more ideas on distracting and pleasurable activities.

In the same way as when you begin to exercise a muscle it is hard work, using this worry time will feel a bit of a challenge at first too. But as you 'exercise the muscle' of controlling your worries, you will become better skilled at keeping your worries under control.

Relaxation training

Progressive muscle relaxation is a form of relaxing in which the major muscle groups in the body are tensed and then relaxed in alternating ways. As everyone holds muscle tension in different parts of their body, progressive muscle relaxation ensures all parts of the body are attended to. It is most helpful to get a CD or an MP3 audio file of someone talking you through the exercise. You will be instructed to start tensing and relaxing the muscles in your feet and then move to your calves, buttocks, thighs, hips, legs, groin, abdomen, hands, forearms, biceps, upper back, shoulders, neck, jaws, eyes and forehead. Each period of muscle tension is held for 5 seconds and then relaxed for 10–15 seconds. Recommended relaxation resources are listed at the end of this chapter.

Controlled breathing

As the anxiety response causes breathing to become more shallow or irregular, controlled breathing can help address this tendency and avoid an imbalance of oxygen and carbon dioxide which can exacerbate the physical symptoms of anxiety further. Simply breathing in to a slow count of 4 and out to a slow count of 4 for three minutes can help you to physically relax.

Imagery

Imagery involves actively visualizing scenes that are relaxing for you. They might be memories of places you have been or know that feel safe, or they may be imagined images that you create in order to feel tranquil. Alternatively you could look through a magazine to find a picture that appeals to you: choose one that invites a feeling of calm and wellbeing. The visual image or memory is important, but do try to incorporate all of your senses: imagine what you would smell and touch and the sounds that might be around you.

References

Butler, Gillian and Hope, Tony (1995). *Manage Your Mind*. Oxford University Press, Oxford.

Hamilton, J. (1995). Needle phobia: a neglected diagnosis. *Journal of Family Practice*, 41(2), 169–75.

Mollema, E., Snoek, F., Pouwer, F., Heine, R. and van der Ploeg, H. (2000) Diabetes fear of injecting and self-testing questionnaire: a psychometric evaluation. *Diabetes Care*, 23(6), 765–9.

Polonsky, William (1999). *Diabetes Burnout*. American Diabetes Association. Alexandria, VA.

Further Reading

Linda Blair (2008). *Straight Talking*. Piatkus, London.

David Burns (1999). *The Feeling Good Handbook*. Random House, New York.

Gillian Butler and Tony Hope (1995). *Manage Your Mind*. Oxford University Press, Oxford.

Dennis Greenberger and Christine Padesky (1995). *Mind Over Mood*. Guilford Press, New York.

Gladeana McMahon (2005). *No More Anxiety: Be Your Own Anxiety Coach*. Karnac Books, London.

William Polonsky (1999). *Diabetes Burnout*. American Diabetes Association, Alexandria, VA.

6

Managing Food, Weight and Emotions

Food and diabetes are inextricably linked. It is hardly surprising, then, that issues with food and eating are commonplace among people with both type 1 and type 2 diabetes. This chapter is not going to give you a plan for losing weight, or offer you any recipes (although there are some recommended resources at the end of the chapter). Instead, it will explain the reasons you may be struggling to fully understand your relationship with food. After setting the scene with some practical issues about food, the chapter is divided into two parts. The first part covers 'emotional eating' – using food to cope with emotions – and how to overcome this. The second part deals with eating disorders, and includes a plan for recovery.

Practical Issues in Managing Eating Behaviour

Increase your knowledge

You may not know where to start with eating well as a person with diabetes. The suggested nutritional guidelines are the same for everyone who is seeking improved health, whether or not you have diabetes. Put simply, food choices that are low in saturated fat and high in fibre, include lots of fruit and vegetables and minimize fat and sugar intake are the best for your health and wellbeing. Eating this way will help you to manage your weight, provide you with more energy and significantly lower your risks for heart disease and cancer. But maybe you are someone who isn't certain

Diabetes and Wellbeing: Managing the Psychological and Emotional Challenges of Diabetes Types 1 and 2,
First Edition. Dr Jen Nash.
© 2013 John Wiley & Sons, Ltd. Published 2013 by John Wiley & Sons, Ltd.

how to translate these guidelines into practical plans. You may well have been provided with advice on healthy eating when you were first diagnosed; however, in the midst of taking in the diagnosis and all its implications, perhaps it was too overwhelming to absorb all the information you were given. Or maybe the guidance was theory-driven (e.g. 'Eat more foods high in fibre') without relating it to practical advice on implementation (e.g. explaining which foods actually contain fibre). You may have felt the stigma and embarrassment that often accompanies diagnosis (see Chapter 3) and had a belief that you should have already known the information you were given, or may not have wanted to risk looking foolish by asking questions to clarify your understanding. Although these are valid and quite natural reactions to dealing with information obtained at diagnosis, the drawback is that your healthcare team may have assumed you had more knowledge than you actually did, making it even more difficult to get the support you now need.

Strive for balance

It is important that you develop a strategy for eating that is clear and reasonable for you, that provides a delicate balance between health and enjoyment. Food is not just fuel for the body, it is one of life's pleasures (more on this later in the chapter). Ideally you will be able, with a member of your healthcare team, to develop a plan for eating that incorporates both health and enjoyment. Following a meal plan that is one hundred per cent healthy one hundred per cent of the time is not realistic for anyone.

Food is a pleasure and it is pretty unrealistic to think that you will never again allow yourself to enjoy the foods that you really love. If your favourite food is apple pie, and you are told that you can never again enjoy it, it is likely that the one thing you will be thinking about, talking about and dreaming about will be apple pie – just because you have been told you cannot have it. Feeling deprived is a problem when it comes to behaviour change: as humans we are designed to seek pleasure and avoid pain and knowing that you can't have something you enjoy is painful! Be flexible and creative about how you can enjoy the foods you love. If you enjoy apple pie, could you see if you can find a supermarket that sells it by the slice? Or create an occasion out of it and go with your friend to have it at a restaurant or coffee shop once a week? Could you spread the fun by having a smaller portion a few times a week instead? Be curious and observe how others around you who seem to stay slim naturally handle eating a wide range of foods. Have a chat with your dietician or diabetes nurse to get their advice on how you can combine a balanced diet with your medication requirements. If, however, you find it difficult to stop eating some types of food once you have started, then the later sections of this chapter will be helpful to you.

Food and your social life

For individuals with diabetes, situations such as restaurants and social events can make maintaining a healthy eating programme more challenging than for others. When you are in social situations you are usually not as in control of your food choices as when you are at home. It can sometimes be difficult to know what is the healthy choice on a restaurant menu. It may take a bit of courage to ask the waiter or waitress to help you out and you may find it embarrassing to do so. You may not know how to ask people what you need in terms of your diabetes.

Further, social events with family and friends can have their own obstacles. Those close to you may need educating about what your needs are in terms of the food they provide. They may have uninformed or outdated assumptions of what you 'should' eat, or they might simply ignore your requests, thinking, 'It's a special occasion, he/she can have a day off' (which you might be able to, but you want that to be your decision, not theirs!). You may feel the tension of wanting to stick to your healthy eating endeavours, but also wanting to enjoy the food the host has prepared. Food is a central part of celebrating, commiserating, and being connected to others in many cultures around the world.

Food is often eaten in social situations and it can be hard to say no to people. One of the reasons you may be uncomfortable saying no is because you do not want to be seen as rude, 'different', or in some way ill or sick because you have got diabetes. Also, you will want to be sensitive to family members for whom food may be a way of conveying their love, care and affection to you. Here are my top three tips for asserting yourself.

Acknowledge you are not being rude   For example if your friend invites you out for ice-cream, you might like to say, 'Thank you for your offer, but I don't eat ice-cream. I hope we can still meet, perhaps for a tea or coffee?' By communicating both parts of the message (by saying I don't want ice-cream and I don't want to hurt your feelings) you can feel more comfortable and confident in what you really mean.

Use 'I' statements   Can you sense the subtle difference between these two responses? 'Thanks. I don't really want any crisps right now' and 'Thanks. Crisps really aren't good for me.' Using 'I' in your statements subtly conveys that you are taking responsibility for your thoughts and feelings. This allows less space for unhelpful responses such as, 'Go on, one won't hurt you!'

Recommend a more suitable action   Shape the behaviour of the person to whom you are responding. If your host is offering you some cake, you could respond with, 'Oh, it looks lovely! I cannot manage any just now but I would like another piece of fruit/cup of tea.' This has two benefits: you are enabling the host to be the host (hosts want to give you something!) and you are also taking control of the interaction, not allowing their agenda to get you off track of yours. Alternatively, you can distract the person with, 'Oh, not for me, thank you; but do tell me about your beautiful/interesting [insert something you have noticed: flowers, painting, dress etc.].'

Now the practical issues with food have been addressed, let's think about the other ways food can be problematic – when it is used to deal with emotions.

Using food to cope with emotions

Do you ever reach the bottom of a packet of crisps or biscuits and wonder how you got there? Or have a bad day at work or an argument with your partner and automatically reach for the ice-cream or a chocolate bar? Perhaps you're someone who needs to or would like to lose weight, and know what you *should* be doing, but can't seem to follow the seemingly simple advice to 'eat more healthily' given by the healthcare professionals you meet, who may also be at a loss to know how to help you.

There are biological, psychological and social reasons why eating well can be so complicated, and many of these reasons overlap to some extent.

Food as a friend   Considering eating has been an inherent part of the survival of our species since time began, there are a great many layers and complexities to the eating process. The important point to understand is that food is not just a source of fuel and energy for the body. The connection between food and emotion is one that is established from birth. From a very young age, food has been intimately linked to your emotions – your mother soothed you with her milk when you were hungry and crying to be fed. As you grew up, the adults in your life gave you sweets to cheer you up after the upset of hurting yourself, or a biscuit when you got in from a hard day at school, or cooked your favourite meal when you had fallen out with a friend. Food is not just a fuel: it has been conditioned as a soother of emotions for as long as you can remember. It is a short cut to good feelings which often happens outside of our awareness, quite unconsciously. Everyone – of every shape and size – can use food to deal with their emotions, and occasionally it can be fine to use food in this way. It is not a problem for the individual who has a wide repertoire of ways to soothe their emotions when needed. The danger is when food becomes the *only* way to deal with emotions.

Everyday life can be stressful. Even without the more intense periods of stress that are inherent in life (like a major life change such as a bereavement, moving house, starting or ending a relationship, birth of a baby, beginning or finishing a job), the ordinary routines of work, family and social obligations require energy to fulfil. Emotions such as sadness, anger, frustration, anxiety, loneliness are also stressful in their own ways. Stress has become such a common ailment of our modern worlds and food is often used as an attempt to deal with it. As an adult, this translates to a 'pull' inside you after a stressful day to reach for some sweet food as a short-cut to those good feelings that you have got through food for as long as you can remember. The physiological response to food is a release of hormones, which means it does act as a limited but effective short-term solution to dealing with stress, probably because when food was scarce it was a stress reliever to find and eat some! When using food to deal with stress, the problem is that the original stressor still remains and using food in this way can add the associated problem of guilt and remorse for the overeating. With two problems to deal with now, and the self-criticism (of being 'weak-willed', etc.) that can come with emotional eating, the original problem is magnified not solved.

When you are diagnosed with diabetes you are suddenly required to begin to focus much more on what (and how much) you are eating. Your healthcare team will encourage you to follow healthier eating regimes, and while you know in your head what you *should* be doing, it is often hard to break away from the pattern of food as a short-cut to pleasure, distraction and satisfaction, and this is rarely discussed in the medical setting.

However, this pattern can be changed. The goal is to reach a place in which you can make a *decision* about whether or not to eat when you are feeling emotional, rather than it just being an automatic response.

The 'good' me versus the 'bad' me   Do you feel that there is a 'good' version of you and a 'bad' version of you, the good version being the one that has a healthy eating plan to follow and knows exactly what you should be doing and when, and the 'bad' version being the little voice inside that says, 'Oh blow it, I deserve to treat myself!'? If this is familiar to you, it is likely that this feels like being on a roller coaster – you are either totally 'on plan' or totally 'off plan'. This often occurs because the 'good' part of your identity around food has a tendency to be overly strict. You may think that you always need to perfectly control your calorie intake and not allow yourself any treats. You therefore may feel you have to be constantly healthy at all times, and may even be feeling hungry some (or a lot) of the time. The problem is that it is incredibly challenging. Remember that food is a source of pleasure and we have been designed to seek out sources of sustenance. In our evolutionary history when food was more likely to be scarce than plentiful, our ancestors would tend to overeat in times of abundance in order to have reserves available in times of shortage. The hunger and appetite centres of the brain are fairly 'unevolved', similar to those of animals, and it is the more evolved part of the brain (called the prefrontal cortex) that is responsible for the more sophisticated thinking, planning and reasoning that needs to kick in to override these primitive desires to nurture. It takes thought and effort to prevail over this instinctual part of you, so go easy on yourself: you are fighting against years of evolution! Having a more thoughtful, compassionate attitude towards yourself that takes into account these two parts of your identity is the ideal way to feeling more in control with your eating. Allowing yourself foods that are pleasurable in a controlled and planned way means you are less likely to 'rebound' and want to devour every sweet/fattening thing in sight if you deviate from an overly rigid plan.

It is hard to resist temptation   In our modern-day society an overwhelming choice and quantity of instantly consumable food is available. We no longer have to seek out, hunt and gather our food: it is on our doorstep. Food is obtainable everywhere and, even with the best intention, it is hard to avoid the constant availability of food. Our environments have changed an incredible amount in a relatively short period of time. It was not so long ago that food was only available to fix the problem it was designed for – to satiate hunger. Now it is ready and available (and packaged accordingly) to be used to solve other problems that it *wasn't* designed to fix, like a bad day at work, frustration with the family or feeling a bit down. Previously, nature provided us with a natural time-delay between thinking about food and being able to eat. Our ancestors would only seek out food when they needed to – they did not use it to solve problems. In contrast you may be sitting on the sofa, find yourself thinking about your stressful day tomorrow, see the bowl of nuts on the coffee table, and your hand is in the bowl almost before you have made the decision to eat.

How to manage emotional eating

Change your world and you change yourself   Your environment plays a hugely important role when you are trying to change your eating habits. Just as in our evolutionary past we had to seek out food, so there was a natural delay between thinking about food and being able to consume it, now it is everywhere we turn! So much of our everyday lives is done habitually, on autopilot. Think of some of your daily routines: how you shower, get to work, what you eat for breakfast. Nine times out of ten you do these in pretty much the same way every day. That is because our brains, as wonderful as they are, have a limited processing capacity and they are designed to create short-cuts to make the demands less arduous. Imagine if you had to concentrate fully on exactly what to do and in which order each time you had a shower!

Spend some time thinking about the ways your environment sabotages you. Perhaps you keep sweets, nuts or chocolates on the coffee table and you find yourself snacking on them while you are watching television in the evenings. Maybe your route home from work is past a fast food restaurant where you can to get a take-away to tide you over until dinnertime. It could be that you have many unhelpful foods in your kitchen at home, so that when you are hungry it is too easy, convenient and tempting to reach for these rather than take a moment to think about an option that might be better for you. Think now about the different environments you find yourself in regularly that sabotage you, and make a note of them here:

Environments that have a tendency to sabotage me

_____

_____

_____

_____

_____

_____

Now you have a clearer sense of the environments that sabotage you, you can start to address them. Rate each on a scale of 0–10, where 0 means it rarely affects you and 10 means it affects you most frequently and most badly. Pick the one that affects you the most to start with, as this will have the greatest impact the quickest. Think about how you can change your environment to support you. Here are some ideas to help you:

Store foods you find tempting out of reach and out of sight (e.g. in the top cupboard of your kitchen rather than on the counter top).

Avoid buying the foods you find tempting in the first place: if they are not at home it takes a lot of effort to get them.

You may want to find a different route home if the food places you pass are too appealing.

If you know a vulnerable time is the evening you may want to rearrange your plans so you're occupied: you could go for a walk or phone a friend.

In restaurants, you could ask the waitress not to bring you the bread bowl, or you could ask for an alternative option to snack on that is lower in calories.

Perhaps you snack while preparing your meals, in which case using pre-prepared vegetables and so on may be an effective way of breaking this habit (you can always return to preparing your own when you have shifted this habit).

Engage in doing something active with your hands, which mean you cannot reach for the food. This could be doing your nails, mending or fixing something, knitting, playing a game on your phone, doing a crossword puzzle, etc.

Remember that there are no rights or wrongs with this process: you are simply making small shifts to the habits you have formed that are no longer truly serving you. Treat it like an experiment: all ideas are good ideas at this stage and you can stop the ones that you do not find helpful and keep the ones you do. Even if you do not make any practical changes right now, just the simple act of gaining insight into how your environment is hindering you is hugely valuable. It enables you to view your situation from a more realistic point of view, showing you the times when you are not at fault, rather your environment is. This helps you to separate some of your tendency for self-criticism and self-blame. If you do continue to eat the snacks on the coffee table, at least you are doing so with your eyes wide open. Knowledge is empowering, and just the increased awareness can translate into different actions over time. Fill in the worksheet below with your own ideas of how your environment triggers you and what changes you can make to help you.

Changes I can make to my environment:

_____

_____

_____

_____

_____

_____

Know the difference between a 'lapse', a 'relapse' and a 'collapse'   Many people embark on weight loss efforts full of enthusiasm and hope for their new regime, and then lose heart when life gets in the way. My advice is different. Embrace the odd slip or two. Actively expect it. Any change in life is usually a process of two steps forward and one step back. In addictions recovery, these backward steps are known as 'lapses', the times when the old, familiar ways of being are the default action we take. Sometimes this is unconscious (for example, your colleague offers you a biscuit with your tea and you take one simply because that is what you have always done).

It is important to be able to distinguish between a lapse, a relapse and a collapse. A lapse is one singular event in which you deviate from your desired goal. An example of a lapse is having a bad day at work or an argument with your partner. You reach for your usual comfort food. crisps or chocolate perhaps, and afterwards, or even while you are still eating, you think, 'Why am I doing this?' That is an example of a lapse. Yes, you have made an unhealthy choice but you can limit it to just one bad decision, get back on track, and continue. A relapse is a whole sequence of lapses strung together. Many people have a very polarized view of success and failure: they are either totally on the plan or totally off it. One lapse becomes, 'I have messed up once so I might as well give up for today.' Then one written-off day can easily become two, until before you know it you are back to where you started. This is a 'collapse'.

The important part is to keep perspective and pay attention to your behaviours over the course of the week, not just focusing on a single day in isolation. Remember that the weight has taken a long time to be part of you, so it is likely to take a long time to lose it. See Chapter 9 for ideas on how to keep focused in the change process.

If you are bored, become less boring!   Food can be very entertaining. It can be a marker between activities and a friend when you are feeling down (even if what you really need is a hug or a listening ear). It can also simply be a convenient form of entertainment if you are feeling bored, restless or fidgety. The first step in overcoming this is simply to become aware that it is a tendency of yours. Know the difference between pleasure and entertainment. All of us find eating pleasurable, but finding entertainment in food is different: it means we are using it to serve a purpose or a function for which another strategy would be better.

If you are lonely, or if there is not much stimulation or excitement in your life, it is common to turn to food for comfort. Food then becomes another problem, while the root problem remains. Taking action on these root causes and addressing your loneliness or boredom is likely to weaken your need to find comfort in food.

Conversely, if you are someone who used to get a lot of enjoyment from food and are now shifting your eating habits and not eating as much 'fun' food any more, you need to find new routes to experiencing fun that do not involve food.

Have a think about the past couple of weeks and consider whether there have been any occasions on which you may have been eating because of boredom or loneliness. Write them here:

Situation and what I was feeling (bored, lonely, etc.)

_____

_____

_____

_____

_____

Now think about how you could start to make changes to this pattern.

Are there any hobbies you used to enjoy? Could you research taking them up again?

Are there old friendships that you could re-establish?

Are there new friends you could make by joining an interest group or organization?

Could you plan a regular coffee shop trip with those in your network?

Are there online groups or internet forums you could find entertainment through?

Could you join an evening class, learn something new and meet new people?

Anything that helps you feel a bit more interested in the world is likely to reduce your cravings for food and the comfort that it can bring.

Deal with emotions directly   Try to pinpoint what emotion you are feeling as you think about reaching for food. The emotion may be positive or negative: anything that stirs up strong feelings can be relevant. Start by labelling it: is it anger, sadness, fury, excitement, hurt, disappointment, excitement, sadness, triumph, boredom, loneliness, shyness, feeling unattractive, worthless? You might like to say to yourself, 'I am – ' and fill in the blank. For example: 'I am [insert emotion] at [insert situation/person/trigger for emotion] because [insert reason].'

Seek out alternative methods for overcoming difficult emotions. Once you build up awareness and self-insight you can really start to feel more in control of your eating behaviours. For instance, you might notice a pattern of reaching for comforting food every Wednesday evening. You realize that on Thursday morning you have a meeting with your boss that you are a bit anxious about. Eating is an attempt to soothe your anxiety about this meeting. Once you have gained an awareness of this try to do something different. You could talk to a supportive friend about ways of expressing yourself differently in the meeting. By being more proactive, you won't necessarily remove the feelings, but you will be doing something much more constructive. Gradually, the urge to binge-eat will become much less compelling.

It's good to talk   Try to reach out to friends and family and let them know about your struggles. As soon as you start to talk about your difficulties with eating, you begin to break down the pattern of secrecy. You can perhaps ask your loved ones to help you, by suggesting activities you could do together in the evening, or helping you to choose healthier options when you go shopping. Gaining support from others close to you is not always possible, however, as sometimes people around you are not ready to change the status quo. In this case, you could see if there are other people you could reach out to for support. Your diabetes clinic, a local meeting of a diabetes charity or an internet resource may be able to connect you to a network of others with diabetes. You can have an informal 'buddy' arrangement to check in with each other every week or month to see how things are going, share ideas, support and encourage each other.

Enjoy being aware of food   Much of the time we eat without really thinking about it or concentrating on the flavours. At meal times you may give more of your attention to watching the television, reading or talking to others than you do to the food itself. Studies have shown that individuals who eat while engaged in other activities consume more that those who are focusing just on their food. Again, eating can happen unconsciously and the calories are not really savoured when you are eating mindlessly in this way. By becoming aware of this and concentrating on your food intake, you can really register the taste, you are more likely to be satisfied and you will probably feel less desire to eat these types of foods in uncontrolled ways.

Try becoming more aware of your food. Choose the food you often binge on and take it with you to a quiet place where there are no distractions. Begin eating in a slow, deliberate way, focusing just on the mouthful you are currently eating. Chew each mouthful thoroughly and really notice the taste, texture and flavours in your mouth. Spend ten minutes a day doing this for a week and see what happens. You will probably find that you are tasting your food a lot more than usual, both in these controlled exercises and at meal times in general. Whilst caught up in a binge, you are likely to eat quickly and frantically, barely even tasting the flavours. Eating in this controlled way, on the other hand, means you are aware of every sensation in your mouth. Visit Chapter 9 on mindfulness techniques to learn more about becoming conscious of your eating.

Also become aware of your habits around food. A very practical strategy is to put a reminder to be aware where you will see it when you reach for food, e.g. a post-it note on the fridge or cupboard, in your bag or wallet. Seeing the note itself may be enough to trigger a different response, or you might like to have a question written directly on the post-it. For example:

Food won't help me with this problem.
The solution is not in here.
Is this what I really want?

Using CBT to Manage Your Emotions Around Food

Case study: Janya

Janya was having a difficult time. She and her partner were arguing a lot and she always felt she was looking after everyone else's needs. The only break she got was when everyone was in bed, and she was struggling to control the amount of food she was eating.

Step 1: What is the situation or event?

Feeling overwhelming emotions just before reaching for food.

Step 2: What do you tell yourself? What are the thoughts you notice running through your mind?

'Life is too hard.'
'I can't manage this.'
'I'm so stressed.'
'To hell with this diet. I deserve a treat'.

Step 3: What is happening in your body and what do you do?

Mood – hopeless, helpless, angry, frustrated
Body sensations – heart beating fast
Behaviours – reach for the food or go to the kitchen to seek some out

Step 4: Challenge your thoughts by asking yourself some helpful questions

What is the evidence for and against this thought?
Is thinking this way helping me?
Are there other ways of thinking about this situation?
If a friend told me they were thinking this way, how would I respond?
Am I thinking in 'all or nothing' terms?
What other points of view are there?
How would someone else think about this?
How else could I think about it?
How would I think about this if I were feeling better?
What are the facts of the case?
How can I find out which way of thinking fits the facts best?
What is the evidence?
Could I be making a mistake in the way I am thinking?
Am I thinking straight?
Am I pressurizing myself?
Am I using the language of the extremist?
What is the worst thing that could happen?

Step 5: Come up with an alternative, balanced thought

'Life is too hard.' Yes, it is. And I can choose to eat, but I know it
   won't solve the real problem; it just gives me another thing to worry
   about. I can choose to do things differently from now on.
'I can't manage this.' Although I don't like struggling with comfort
   eating, I like other parts of my life, like my relationship with the
   kids and my job. I am learning to control my eating.
'I'm so stressed.' I have a right to feel this anger/upset /frustration.
   Food won't change that, it will only complicate the situation with a
   new feeling.
'To hell with this diet. I deserve a treat.' I do deserve a 'treat' but it
   does not have to be food. I can choose to think of other ways to
   treat myself, e.g. have a bubble bath or watch a DVD.

After having done this exercise, you may still go ahead and eat the
food. If you do, do not beat yourself up for this! Change takes time,
and simply by pausing and thinking about the reasons behind your
actions involving food you are making a great start. At least if you
eat this time you will be making a deliberate choice to do so, rather
than feeling like you are acting as if you had no control over your
behaviour.

Use a kindness statement

Turn your alternative thought into a kindness statement to remind
yourself of in the times when you are tempted to binge-eat. This is to
be read three times a day at least, and also left in the places when you
are most likely to binge, for example on a sticky note in the kitchen.

Learn to relax

Once you have read your kindness statement, you might like to think
of some other way to soothe or dissipate the unwanted emotions.
Sometimes food can be used as a way to provide an energy boost when
rest is what is really needed. You might want to have a lie-down or
a nap, or try a relaxation CD or podcast. Some of these simply have
soothing music, others have someone guiding you through a specific
relaxation exercise.

Talk to your healthcare team

Finally, next time you are having a conversation about your weight with a member of your healthcare team, perhaps you could share this book with them and have a discussion about the emotional reasons that you sometimes eat. Breaking out of the secrecy tied up in comfort eating is one of the most important things you can do. By becoming aware of your emotions you can see that they have evolved to support and guide you. With time, emotions can become your friend rather than an enemy to be dulled with food.

Diabetes and Eating Disorders

What are eating disorders?

As we have seen, eating behaviour is rarely straightforward. But what turns difficulties with food into an eating disorder? Put simply, an eating disorder is diagnosed if your attitude towards food causes you to change your eating habits and behaviours in a way that may cause damage to your health. The most common eating disorders are:

Anorexia nervosa: when someone tries to keep their weight as low as possible, for example by starving themselves or exercising excessively.

Bulimia nervosa: when someone binge-eats and then tries to control their weight by deliberately being sick or using laxatives, diuretics and enemas.

Eating disorder not otherwise specified: an eating disorder that does not meet the criteria for any specific eating disorder. This includes binge eating disorder, when someone feels compelled to overeat but doesn't use any compensatory behaviours (such as self-induced vomiting, laxatives, diuretics or enemas).

One type of eating disorder not otherwise specified (EDNOS) that is specific to people with diabetes who use insulin is the reduction or omission of insulin. This behaviour is often referred to as 'diabulimia' in the media, although most health professionals avoid this term because it is confusing on many fronts: for instance, bulimia involves making yourself sick, which many individuals with diabetes who manipulate insulin do not do.

EDNOS-DMT1 (diabetes mellitus type 1) is a preferable term, although the condition is not clinically recognized yet. With insulin omission, whether by decreasing, delaying, or completely omitting prescribed insulin doses, a person with diabetes can induce hyperglycaemia and rapidly lose calories in the urine in the form of glucose.

Insulin manipulation can be done in quite a secretive way, so it often goes undetected by healthcare professionals. Unfortunately, it can also easily be misunderstood and the patient labelled 'non-compliant' with treatment. However, individuals who are manipulating their insulin are struggling with an eating disorder.

Signs to look out for that may suggest insulin omission

Recurrent episodes of diabetic ketoacidosis (DKA)/hyperglycaemia
High HbA1c
Frequent hospitalizations for poor blood sugar control
Delay in puberty or sexual maturation, or irregular periods
Frequent trips to the toilet
Frequent episodes of thrush/urine infections
Nausea and stomach cramps
Loss of appetite
Eating more but losing weight
Drinking an abnormal amount of fluids
Delayed healing from infections/ bruises
Easy bruising
Dehydration and dry skin
Dental problems
Blurred vision
Severe fluctuations in weight
Fractures/bone weakness
Anaemia and other deficiencies
Early onset of diabetic complications, particularly neuropathy, retinopathy, gastroperisis and nephropathy
Anxiety/distress over being weighed at appointments
Fear of hypoglycaemia
Fear of injecting/extreme distress at injecting
Injecting in private/out of view
Avoidance of diabetes-related health appointments
Lack of blood glucose testing/reluctance to test

Are you currently struggling with an eating disorder?

You may well recognize some of the signs in the list above. The Diabetes Eating Problems Scale–Revised (Markowitz, Butler, Volkening et al., 2010) is a self-report questionnaire that allows you to measure your current experiences of anxiety. Answer the questions in Box 6.1 as they relate to your experience.

Box 6.1 Do you have an eating disorder?

Diabetes Eating Problems Scale-Revised (Markowitz, Butler, Volkening et al., 2010)

1. Losing weight is an important goal to me.
2. I skip meals and/or snacks.
3. Other people have told me that my eating is out of control.
4. When I overeat, I don't take enough insulin to cover the food.
5. I eat more when I am alone than when I am with others.
6. I feel that it's difficult to lose weight and control my diabetes at the same time.
7. I avoid checking my blood sugar when I feel like it is out of range.
8. I make myself vomit.
9. I try to keep my blood sugar high so that I will lose weight.
10. I try to eat to the point of spilling ketones in my urine.
11. I feel fat when I take all of my insulin.
12. Other people tell me to take better care of my diabetes.
13. After I overeat, I skip my next insulin dose.
14. I feel that my eating is out of control.
15. I alternate between eating very little and eating huge amounts.
16. I would rather be thin than have good control of my diabetes.

Questions are scored on a 6-point scale:

0   never
1   rarely
2   sometimes
3   often
4   usually
5   always

A score of 20 or more indicates an eating problem. So what have you discovered? Perhaps you are not currently experiencing any or many eating disorder symptoms at all, in which case you can move ahead to another chapter, or read the information that follows as a reference in case your situation changes in the future. Or maybe you are at the other extreme, and your score demonstrates that you are struggling with significantly disordered eating currently. Wherever you are, the following sections will help you to understand why you are feeling this way and how to get better.

Causes of eating disorders

Causes of eating disorders are complex, and there is rarely one specific cause. Rather, as with other emotional difficulties there are biopsychosocial reasons for their development and continuation. The reasons that disordered eating may develop in the general population (i.e. non diabetes-specific reasons) are:

Biological

Having a family history of eating disorders, depression or substance misuse
Being female (although men are also increasingly vulnerable and do also develop eating disorders)
Being overweight
Experiencing early puberty compared to peers.

Psychological

Being overly concerned with being slim, particularly if combined with pressure to be slim from society or for a job (which can happen, for example, to ballet dancers, models or athletes)
Certain characteristics, for example having an obsessive personality, an anxiety disorder or low self-esteem, or being a perfectionist
Dietary restraint and dieting.

Social

being criticized for one's eating habits, body shape or weight
particular experiences, such as sexual or emotional abuse or the death of someone special
difficult relationships with family members or friends

stressful situations, for example problems at work, school or university
disturbed family functioning
disturbed parental eating attitudes
peer and cultural influences.

Eating disorders are often blamed on the social pressure to be thin. However, although this can be a contributing factor for some individuals, the causes are usually more complex: many people do feel a pressure to be slim but do not go on to develop an eating disorder.

If you are struggling with an eating disorder it is not your fault. You are likely to have difficulty in managing and regulating your emotions, and a distorted view of your own body image. You are concerned about your body weight and shape and are likely to believe that you are overweight when you are actually at a normal or low weight. You probably fear gaining weight or becoming fat, and have a concerned attitude towards food, calories and eating. Thoughts about food, weight and shape are likely to be on your mind much of the time, and your success in controlling your eating behaviour and weight can become a main way you feel good about yourself.

Eating disorders and type 1 diabetes

Considerable evidence has also accumulated to suggest that living with type 1 diabetes in itself is a risk factor for disturbed eating behaviour and eating disorders (Nielsen, 2002). Eating disorders have been found to be twice as common in teenage girls with type 1 diabetes as in their peers without diabetes (Colton, Rodin, Bergenstal and Parkin, 2009). It is also argued that the diabetes treatment goals can 'teach' or intensify some of the vulnerability to an eating disorders mindset (Goebel-Fabbri, 2009).

Diabetes management increases the focus on controlled food intake, and can be experienced as restrictive. This means you are following an eating plan which is not completely dependent on responding to your own internal cues for hunger and fullness. This results in these cues becoming less reliable. If you undereat you are likely to feel deprived, which can trigger overeating and binge eating episodes. Knowing that bingeing is not good for your health or weight, you may then intensify your efforts to control your food intake and weight, getting trapped in a cycle of dieting, further binge eating, and weight control behaviour.

Not only this, but at puberty, when weight and shape concerns intensify, diabetes can become more difficult to manage due to hormonal changes and resulting insulin resistance. Diabetes then may constitute a pathway of risk for the development of disturbed eating behaviour.

Insulin manipulation or omission　　Insulin manipulation is the most common method of purging in girls with type 1 diabetes and becomes progressively more common through the teen years. This behaviour is reported by 2% of pre-teen girls, 11–15% of girls in the mid-teen years and 30–39% of those in the late teenage and early adult years (Colton, Rodin, Bergenstal and Parkin, 2009).

The reason most frequently cited by women with type 1 diabetes for deliberate insulin omission is weight control. However, other motivating factors may include:

fear of hypoglycaemia
denial of having diabetes
embarrassment about blood glucose testing or insulin administration in
    front of others
desire to have a break from diabetes management
fear of needles
secondary weight gain

These additional factors are addressed in more detail in other chapters of this book. They can operate in combination with a desire to control weight to worsen and entrench the insulin omission behaviour.

Eating disorders and type 2 diabetes

In individuals with type 2 diabetes, binge eating disorder appears to be the most common eating disorder (Herpertz, Albus, Lichtblau et al., 2000). It has been suggested that the diagnosis and management of type 2 diabetes generally does not worsen or precipitate an eating disorder, but eating disorders, predominantly binge eating disorder, are more likely to be found among those with type 2 diabetes because of the association of both conditions with being overweight.

Overcoming an eating disorder

If you are currently struggling with an eating disorder then I want to praise you for reading this chapter. Being able to be honest with yourself and admit that you are having difficulties with eating is an important first step in the journey of recovery. Whatever eating issue you have, I encourage you to gain support from someone else, by telling a family member, trusted friend, or health professional. Struggling alone is hard and one of the most important steps forward (although sometimes also the hardest) is to admit how you feel to someone else. If you do not feel ready to do that yet, then work through the material that follows in this chapter. Hopefully, by reading about the process of change you will be encouraged to consider the next step you could take.

As bulimia, binge eating and insulin omission are the most common eating disorders that affect people with diabetes, the treatment approaches described in this chapter will focus on these disorders. If you are struggling with anorexia, much of this information will still be relevant for you, but you will need some additional support to increase your food intake. Please see the recommended resources at the end of the chapter for further details.

Although biological treatments using antidepressants are sometimes warranted to treat the depression that can accompany an eating disorder, this chapter will focus on the psychological and social ways of addressing disordered eating, outlining the 10 steps to overcoming an eating disorder. Start at step A and work your way through the steps methodically if you can, obviously skipping any that is not relevant for you (for example, step C, developing an eating plan, can be ignored if you are not currently omitting insulin). However, if you are feeling overwhelmed, start at whichever step feels most possible. Any step towards recovery is important progress.

Ten steps to overcoming your eating disorder

A. Get ready to change
B. Keep a diary
C. Develop an insulin/food plan
D. Reduce binge eating
E. Reduce vomiting/laxative use
F. Examine your thinking
G. Problem-solve
H. Expect challenges
 I. Increase self-esteem
J. Speak up

Step A: Get ready to change

The first step in overcoming an eating disorder is becoming willing to change. By reading this far, you are demonstrating you are somewhat ready to at least contemplate change. Perhaps you have had enough and are desperate to change, or maybe you are a bit more unsure; your behaviour around food, although not ideal, does bring you some advantages. Let's clarify your readiness to change. Take two pieces of paper. On one piece write 'Reasons to give up the eating disorder' and on the other write 'Reasons not to give up the eating disorder'. Being able to see the reasons both for and against in black and white is helpful. You might want to divide your thinking up in terms of the things you gain and lose, both practically and emotionally, for yourself and in relation to others.

Case study: Juliet

Reasons to give up binge eating
Practical advantages that relate to myself
I won't have to spend so much money on food.
I will look healthier.
My diabetes will be better controlled and I will be healthier.

Practical advantages that relate to others
I will be less irritable.
I will be a better employee and colleague at work – less distracted.
I won't eat food that belongs to others.

Emotional advantages that relate to myself
I will feel I have achieved something.
I can stop lying.

Emotional advantages that relate to others
My family will stop worrying about my health.
I can join in with social activities.
My boss will be pleased that I'm not sneaking off all the time (to eat).

Disadvantages to changing binge eating

Practical disadvantages that relate to myself

I am worried I will put on more weight if I eat regularly.
I will find meal times with others difficult.

Practical disadvantages that relate to others

I might be moodier if I can't binge to help me cope.
I might cry more.

Emotional disadvantages that relate to myself

I will feel out of control with everything.
It will be difficult and I am bound to fail, making me feel worse about
   myself.

Emotional disadvantages that relate to others

If others find out that I have a problem with binge eating they may be
   ashamed of me.
If I'm more moody or cry more I might change, and others may not
   like me as much.

Reasons to change

Practical advantages that relate to myself

1.
2.
3.

Practical advantages that relate to others

1.
2.
3.

Emotional advantages that relate to myself

1.
2.
3.

Emotional advantages that relate to others
1.
2.
3.

Disadvantages to changing binge eating

Practical disadvantages that relate to myself
1.
2.
3.

Practical disadvantages that relate to others
1.
2.
3.

Emotional disadvantages that relate to myself
1.
2.
3.

Emotional disadvantages that relate to others
1.
2.
3.

Do not rush this list – come back to it each day over a week to review it and see if any other reasons have come up for you. Once you have finished, go over the list and rate each reason on a scale of 1–10, where 10 signifies a very important reason and 1 signifies an only slightly important reason.

Once you have done this, you can use it to complete an activity called 'Back to the Future' (from Schmidt and Treasure, 2007). Imagine yourself in five years' time, after you had decided it was too difficult and risky to overcome your eating disorder. You continue to have disordered eating. Everything has gone wrong. All the negative consequences that you considered in your balance sheet have come true. You feel at the end of your tether. You decide to write to your one close friend, whom you haven't seen for a while as she (assuming she is a woman) has been abroad. You know that she cares about you and will not be deceived by superficial news and that when you meet her on her return she will see it all anyway. You have found in the past that she has been able to provide emotional and practical support when you have needed help. You know that you can, and must, give her a full account of your present difficulties.

Here are a few guidelines to consider:

What weight will you be?
What medical complications will you have?
What career/job will you be pursuing?
Where and with whom will you be living?
Who will be your friends?
Will you be in a relationship? Married? Have children?

Now be as realistic as possible, and talk in the present tense as you write your letter below.

First letter to my future self

```



```

Once you have written your own letter, read it through. Does this sound like a future you want?

Now write a second letter, again imagining your situation in five years' time, except this time you have successfully recovered from your eating disorder. Read this through – how does that sound?

Second letter to my future self

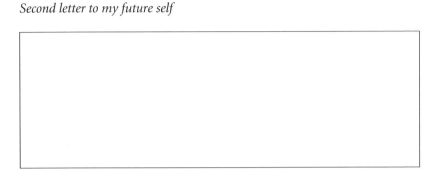

Doing this exercise may have inspired you to throw yourself fully into recovery – in which case, good for you! It is important to be realistic though. Many people state, 'I'm never going to binge again in my life', which is going to be hard to maintain. After all, you have developed this behaviour over time, and it will take time to recover. Small and steady steps in the right direction are much more achievable.

Once you have made a decision to recover – congratulations! Set aside time at least once a week (more often if you can) in which you can review how you're doing, read this book and see where you've got to in terms of your goals.

Step B: Keep a diary

One of the most important aspects to changing difficulties with eating and insulin behaviour is to get a clear picture of your current situation. The best way to do this is to keep track of everything you eat and drink for a week, and the accompanying behaviours (such as self-induced vomiting) or absence of behaviours (such as having less insulin than you need). This can feel like a big job at first, so try and go easy on yourself. Start it on a day when you know life will be quiet and do not despair if you only manage to keep it for a couple of days in the first week; this is all progress. Use bullet points and abbreviations to help. To help with accuracy, carry your diary with you and try and complete it as the day is happening, rather than all at the end. If using a detailed diary of the kind shown in Table 6.1 feels too overwhelming, you can do the diary in stages, by making a note of what you eat for a week (perhaps in your phone) until you get into the habit of it. Then you can move on to the more detailed approach (Table 6.2).

Table 6.1 Example diary

When and where was I?	What was I doing? Who was I with?	What I ate and drank	Binge? Yes/No	Behaviour: vomit (V), laxatives (L), exercise (E), insulin (I) or omission (IO)?	Triggers What started it? Reason for behaviour? Thoughts What went through my mind (before and after the behaviour)? Feelings Physical sensations and emotions (before and after the behaviour)
7.30 Kitchen	Deciding what to eat for breakfast. Alone	Cereal	No	IO	Want to get into my dress for my date on Friday night – need to lose a few pounds.
12.30 College canteen	With friends	Soup	No	IO	Really wanted the chips my friends were eating
3 pm On way home	After college. Alone	3 doughnuts, 4 chocolate bars, large milkshake	Yes	V	Felt rubbish about my work and wanted to forget the day. Afterwards, felt disgusted with myself

Table 6.2 Your diary

When and where was I?	What was I doing? Who was I with?	What I ate and drank	Binge? Yes/No	Behaviour: vomit (V), laxatives (L), exercise (E), insulin (I) or omission (IO)?	**Triggers** What started it? Reason for behaviour? **Thoughts** What went through my mind (before and after the behaviour)? **Feelings** Physical sensations and emotions (before and after the behaviour)

Step C: Establish an insulin routine that feels achievable

If you are currently taking less insulin than you should, then I want to talk to you, not as a health professional, but as a young woman with diabetes who has also struggled with her body image. I do not want you to hear this as a lecture, as that is not my intention. I hope that you will read this in a spirit of openness, that if you have read this far you are open to change. I know that taking less insulin than your body needs has payoffs to you. You like feeling slim and being able to eat what you like. However, just as you would not survive long without oxygen or water, your body cannot survive without insulin. If you are going more than a day without insulin, it is critical that you start to give yourself some insulin each day, no matter how small. Every unit you can give yourself is helping you stay alive. Being thin is not worth losing your life over (if you think it is, then I strongly urge you to read my advice in Chapter 3 on what to do if you are feeling suicidal). You are a unique person who deserves health, even if you do not see that in yourself right now. At the end of the chapter are listed some organizations where you can access support from others who have been where you are and recovered.

I also need to talk to you about how to keep yourself safe. You are at high risk from diabetic ketoacidosis (DKA), which can cause death. The signs of DKA are shown below. If you develop these symptoms you must seek urgent medical help, either by taking yourself to hospital or calling 999.

nausea and vomiting
dehydration
dry mouth
pronounced thirst
excessive urine production
abdominal pain
hyperglycaemia on blood glucose testing
confusion

Take a look at your diary and notice how much insulin you have been giving yourself each day, or each week if there are some days when you are not having any insulin at all. Set yourself a goal to increase the quantity in small amounts each day. If there are some days when you are not injecting at all, aim to establish a routine in which you can inject your basal (long-acting) insulin every day of the week.

Step D: Reduce binge eating

Why do you binge   There are both physical and psychological reasons for binge eating. You may find you are struggling with just one of these reasons, or many of them.

The physical reasons for binge eating are that, if you are eating less than you need (through dieting, for example), your body is designed to alert you through cravings that it is not receiving enough nutrition. If you do binge, and then cut out meals in the hours that follow to make up for having eaten too much, you are 'programming' the next binge. When you have used alcohol or drugs you may also be more prone to a binge, as these substances reduce your inhibitions and resolve.

The psychological and emotional reasons arise from the fact that, as eating can be comforting, an impulse to binge can occur in relation to feeling stress, tension, anxiety, boredom, loneliness or depression. If you are someone who likes to feel in control, and have a high degree of perfectionism, then any deviation from your usual eating plan can trigger a binge (evident in the thought 'I've failed now anyway, I might as well carry on'.).

In the same way as there are both physical and psychological reasons for a binge, there are both physical and psychological strategies for overcoming the urge to binge. Here are some recommended do's and don'ts to tackle your binge eating:

Do:

aim to eat more regular meals (and with planned, regular snacks in between if you can) to reduce strong cravings for food

even if you binge, eat your next planned meal as usual

try to limit your binges to just one place

try to restrict your bingeing to just part of the day

write a list of situations that trigger your binges and find ways of dealing with them (e.g., being alone, feeling anxious about something, wearing certain clothes)

anticipate danger zones, e.g. weekends with a lot of unstructured time. Draw up a timetable of pleasurable activities for the weekend and stick to it

when you get the urge to binge, distract yourself by doing something that is incompatible with bingeing, like going for a walk, phoning or seeing a friend, tidying a drawer

have a planned binge (see below)

get in touch with others (see recommended resources) and find out what
   helped them
avoid people, places and things that are associated with bingeing for you.

Don't:

shop for food when you are hungry
blame yourself if you've had a binge. Instead look at what led up to the
   behaviour so you can learn something for next time
weigh yourself more frequently than once a week: weight fluctuates naturally
   from day to day.

Step E: Reduce vomiting/laxative use

The next step is to tackle any behaviour that you are using to attempt to
purge yourself of food that you have consumed, such as vomiting, or using
laxatives, diuretics or enemas. Reducing these behaviours is likely to make
you feel very anxious, so there are some ideas for how to manage this at the
end of this step.

Look at your diary and work out the average time that you let elapse
between eating and using a purging behaviour. Over the next week, each
day try to delay the purging for this length of time until your anxiety at
delaying subsides. Once you can do this most days, move on to a longer
interval (perhaps by five minutes, or longer if you can).

If you always vomit straight after eating, start by delaying for just five
minutes and increase this over the days. It is better to start small and achieve
success than fail immediately because of a goal that is too challenging.

If your diary shows that you use a purging behaviour less than four times
a week, then instead your aim is to use your purging once less often this
week than last week. Continue cutting down every week or every other
week until you have stopped.

How to cope with your anxiety   Cutting down on your purging behaviour
in this way will make you feel very anxious, and you will be full of fear of
gaining weight. Distraction is the best strategy for riding out this anxiety.
Ideas for distraction are:

Talk to someone (in person or on the phone)
Go for a walk
Clear out a cupboard

Organize a day out
Do a craft, e.g. sewing, making a card, fixing or repairing something
Do a crossword or puzzle
Paint your nails
Pray
Write a letter to a friend

See other ideas for distraction in the list of pleasurable activities in Chapter 4.

Step F: Examine your thinking

Just as in other areas covered in this book, skills drawn from cognitive behavioural therapy (CBT) can help to tackle some of your unhelpful thinking about your eating, your weight and other aspects of yourself in relation to your body image.

Using CBT in Relation to Eating, Weight and Body Image

Case study: Harriet

Harriet is skipping her insulin. She started doing it just occasionally, when she wanted to lose weight for a date, but now she does it most days and she is scared of putting on weight. She knows that this is not healthy but has mixed feelings about changing.

Case study: Dinishia

Dinishia has been bingeing and making herself sick most days. She has found out that she has not got into her university of choice and is now going to be staying at home for a year while her friends move on with their lives.

Step 1: What is the situation or event?

Harriet   Knowing that I need insulin but not having any.
Dinishia   Feeling a compulsion to binge.

Step 2: What do you tell yourself? What are the thoughts you notice running through your mind?

Harriet

If I lose a stone, my life will be OK.
If I was slim people would like me more.
I'm no use. I'm so fat and ugly.
I need to feel in control.

Dinishia

I'm worthless. I'm so fat and ugly I might as well have a binge.
I'm rubbish at everything. The only comfort I have is in food.
No one loves or cares about me.

Step 3: What is happening in your body and what do you do?

Harriet

Mood – fearful, anxious.
Body sensations – heart beating fast, feel on edge all the time.
Behaviours – pretend to go to the bathroom to inject when I'm with
    others.

Dinishia

Mood – hopeless and helpless, angry at myself.
Body sensations – feel 'slowed down'.
Behaviours – reach for the food or seek some out.

Step 4: Challenge your thoughts by asking yourself some helpful questions

What is the evidence for and against this thought?
Is thinking this way helping me?
Are there other ways of thinking about this situation?
If a friend told me they were thinking this way, how would I respond?
Am I thinking in 'all or nothing' terms?

What other points of view are there?
How would someone else think about this?
How else could I think about it?
How would I think about this if I were feeling better?
What are the facts of the case?
How can I find out which way of thinking fits the facts best?
What is the evidence?
Could I be making a mistake in the way I am thinking?
Am I thinking straight?
Am I pressurizing myself?
Am I using the language of the extremist?
What is the worst thing that could happen?

Step 5: Come up with an alternative, balanced thought
Harriet

'If I lose a stone my life will be OK.' My life would still have the same difficulties if I lost weight. That would not change the problems.
'If I was slim people would like me more.' I know that I like people of all different shapes and sizes. Why would other people be any different?
'I'm no use. I'm so fat and ugly.' I may feel that I am fat and ugly but that does not mean that I am no use. I have managed to keep going to work despite my problems. I do have some value.
'I want to feel in control.' I do like to feel in control, but life cannot be completely controlled and learning to tolerate a bit of disorder is an important life skill. Although I do not like the feeling of being out of control, it cannot hurt me.
I have a right to feel these feelings. Food won't change that. It will only complicate the situation with a new feeling.

Dinishia

'I'm worthless. I'm so fat and ugly I might as well have a binge.' I may feel that I am worthless but that does not mean I *am* worthless. I managed to comfort my friend when she broke up with her boyfriend.

'I'm rubbish at everything. The only comfort I have is in food.' I feel
a bit rubbish but I do get comfort from stroking my cat and from
having a hot bubble bath.
'No one loves or cares about me.' I know my mum and sister do love
me. And my friends. It's me that doesn't always care about me.
I have a right to feel angry, upset and frustrated that I haven't got into
the university I wanted to. I can express this through punching a
pillow for five minutes every day, writing or drawing how I feel, and
talking about how I feel to my mum.

Step G: Learn how to problem-solve

If you have an eating disorder, it is likely that you have used it to help you
cope with, or avoid or escape from, some of the difficulties you experience
in life. It is important then to develop some new skills to help you solve
some of life's problems more directly. Here is a seven-step process for more
effective problem solving (Schmidt and Treasure, 2007).

1. What is your problem? Write it in one sentence.

2. What are the solutions? Brainstorm every conceivable solution you can
come up with, even if it seems unrealistic or silly. The idea is to think of as
many as possible.

3. Look at all the options in detail? Go through the pros and cons of each
possible solution.

4. Choose a solution that suits you By examining the pros and cons you
can probably see that there are one or two that best suit you.

5. Plan to implement your solution Think through all the steps you need
to take, and in which order, to implement the solution.

6. Carry it out step by step It may feel hard to do, but stick with it, as you
are learning a new skill for life.

7. Review the outcome Once you have implemented the solution, review
it to learn for next time. Knowing what you know now, would you have
chosen a different solution?

Step H: Expect challenges

One thing is for sure as you tackle your eating disorder: you will have slip-ups and lapses. It is important to prepare for these and to actively expect them. They do not mean you are a failure. Just as an infant learning to walk falls down countless times before she masters it, you too are learning a new way of being. Although you may want to avoid thinking about your lapses, try to examine them so you can learn from them for next time. Here are some questions to ask yourself about a slip-up.

Was it caused by stress, guilt, reward, upset, anxiety, unhappiness, excitement, or any other feeling? If so, what other ways of dealing with these triggers do you have?

Is eating still the easiest and quickest way of getting pleasure or a break in your life? If so, are there changes you can make so that you have a variety of routes to pleasure or a break from the demands of life?

It can be tempting to ignore or avoid your lapses because of shame and guilt. However, if you can look at them you can learn from them, which will help you to cope differently next time. For instance, if stress is a trigger and you have a stressful event coming up tomorrow, you could plan to meet a friend or engage in some enjoyable activity. Alternatively, you may continue to binge for a time, but at least if you've examined your behaviour you will be doing so with insight, in a 'knowing' way, rather than in an unconscious or confused fashion. Remember, although it may seem to come out of the blue, there is *always* a reason for a binge; it just needs to be found.

Take control of your slip-ups by planning one   Set aside some time when you will not be disturbed. Buy all your favourite binge foods and lay them out on the table in front of you. As you begin to eat, concentrate on the process as much as you can. Notice if anything has shifted, either in the amount or in the way you are eating it. It is likely to, because it was planned and you therefore had a greater sense of control over the experience. You could have a planned binge each week, decreasing it to once a fortnight, once a month, and so on.

Physical challenges to recovery   If you have been omitting insulin, your body may develop some short-term physical symptoms as balance is restored and your health returns. It is upsetting to experience these, but for some they are an unfortunate part of recovery. Remember they are short-term, and once you have got through them you will be feeling so much better in your health. Just as the athlete needs to endure injuries, muscle ache and fatigue to reach her goal, so these physical symptoms are short-term pains for long-term gain.

As your body returns to normal you may experience fluid retention, which makes you feel fat, bloated and uncomfortable. This is *not* the development of fat tissue and is temporary (it is similar to the fluid retention that many women experience in relation to their menstrual cycle). Ensure that you drink enough fluids, and limit your intake of caffeine (in tea, coffee, cola and chocolate). You may also experience symptoms of gastroparesis, such as bloating, nausea and excessive fullness. Medications are available to treat this, so do go to your GP or pharmacist for advice. Peripheral neuropathy may also worsen in the short term as your diabetes control improves.

Although these symptoms are unfair, they are short-term. Through recovery, you will feel better than you have done in a long time. I encourage you to get support from others who have negotiated the recovery journey successfully. Please see the recommended resources at the end of the chapter for sources of support.

Step I: Increase self-esteem

Eating disorders can destroy self-esteem, because of the guilt and shame that are often tied up in the behaviour. Yes, you have an eating disorder, but you still have worth as a person. You may have got a sense of esteem from managing to control your weight or your eating behaviours, and this may be threatened as you recover. I would like you to think about other, non-food and non-weight routes to self-esteem.

Create a record of your achievements   Write down (or draw if you prefer) everything you have accomplished in your life. Review the list daily and add new ideas to it as often as you can. If you find it difficult and hear yourself wondering what you have achieved, think about what others have said to you, or even ask someone close to you what qualities they admire in you.

Case study: Geeta's record of achievements   At first Geeta found it difficult to think of anything. But over a few days she managed to come up with the following list.

Learned how to use a computer
I am a good sister
Passed my A-levels
Can play the guitar
People tell me I'm good at putting fashion outfits together

I'm organized
I like my smile
I planned a successful surprise party for my friend
I can tell a couple of good jokes that make people laugh

Engage in activities that make you feel good about yourself   Are there
activities, interests or parts of your identity that have made you feel good
about yourself that you could try again? A particular hobby or craft,
complimenting others, doing something nice for someone, getting in touch
with your spiritual side or spending time with animals.

Case study: Geeta   Geeta really enjoyed horse riding when she was younger
but had not been for years. Although she was not sure if she could spend
the money on it now, she decided she would look on the internet and find
out: she could always save up or ask her family members to club together
for her birthday. She also knew of a field locally where there was a footpath
close by where she could stand and stroke the horses. Just being near horses
seemed to lift her spirits slightly and make her feel a bit better about things.

Diary of everyday successes   Keep a diary of everyday achievements and
record at least three each day. These can be food- or diabetes-related or
not, as you can see from Geeta's diary.

Case study: Geeta's diary of everyday successes

1. I went to work even though I didn't feel like it.
2. I managed to give myself two units more insulin today than yesterday.
3. I saw the horses and they made me feel a bit better.

Be less perfect and overcome shame   Often low self-esteem can be difficult to
tackle because the person with an eating disorder has a need to be or feel 'perfect' (however you define this), and anything less than this is just not acceptable. Often a need for perfectionism develops in response to a need to feel in
control of things: when other parts of your life are feeling out of control (and
it is hard to think of any aspect of life that we can control completely), being
able to control your weight, shape and food intake can help bring relief.
Feelings of shame, embarrassment and humiliation are closely linked to the
idea that you must be perfect or else nobody will like you. To beat these
feelings you could increase your tolerance for being less perfect. Ideas are:

Drop something in public.
Wear odd socks.

Walk into a local shop with a small pen line drawn on your face.

Don't wear any (or wear less) make-up for a day.

Have a hole in your jumper or tights.

Deliberately let something small go wrong at work.

Tell someone about an embarrassing event, e.g. tripping up or spilling something.

Dress comfortably at a formal event.

Pretend you do not have enough money to pay for your shopping at the checkout till.

Tell someone you trust about your eating issues.

Step J: Speak up

Many people with eating disorders have a tendency to like to please others, to put others' needs before their own, and to find it difficult to say no. Tired and worn out from meeting others' needs, the only respite they find is through the comfort and soothing of food, or through controlling it. Increasing your assertiveness, to be confident in your self-esteem and value, to be able to prioritize your needs as well as others', is an important skill to develop. The first step is to know the difference between passive, assertive and aggressive styles of communication.

Passive: Your own wants, needs and feelings are silenced. Typical phrases of passivity are: 'I wonder if you could possibly . . . ?'; 'It's all right, don't worry about it'; 'maybe'.

Assertive: You express your own wants, needs and feelings, but also take into account the feelings of the person to whom you are talking.

Aggressive: You only consider your own wants, needs and feelings. Emotions are expressed inappropriately, with anger or hostility.

Being passive is often the most familiar, and if this is the style you regularly engage it you may find yourself suddenly swinging to being aggressive and expressing yourself angrily, and then feeling remorse for this. Assertiveness is the more challenging territory to find.

Not being assertive leads to a gradual build-up of frustration which will keep your eating problems going. Ignoring conflict with others can be tempting, but it is only a short-term solution. Over time frustration will increase, and it's easier in the long term to deal with potential conflicts as they arise.

How to be assertive

Plan in advance what you want to achieve and any possible responses that might come up.

Choose your timing. Often a time when you are alone with the person is best.

Make eye contact. If you find eye contact challenging, practise maintaining it with yourself in the mirror and then with family members or friends. When you get the urge to break away, challenge yourself to hold it for just a second or two more, and build up from there.

Be specific and direct in your request: 'Can you help me with this please?' rather than, 'I'm sorry to bother you but I was just wondering if you could possibly consider giving me a hand.'

If you need to criticize, focus on the behaviour, not the person. Give the negative feedback sandwiched between positive statements: 'I really enjoy working for you, but I feel frustrated when I am expected to work late without any notice. I want to mention it as I like the job and I do want to be flexible.'

When you have to say no, suggest alternatives (but only if you want to): 'I'm afraid I can't stay late at work this evening as I have plans; however, I could do tomorrow if that is helpful to you.'

Use the broken record technique. If the person tries to convince you of their point of view, repeat your point (e.g. 'I am not able to work late today'), calmly, time after time if need be, or change the subject.

You have permission to change your mind. If you have second thoughts about something you have agreed to, you can simply say, 'I'm sorry but I will not be able to do ___ after all'. It is your life, and you have a right to put your needs first.

In preparation for a difficult conversation:

- Write down brief notes of what you would like to say.
- Practise how you would like to express this in front of the mirror.
- Audio or video yourself on your mobile phone and listen to or watch it back.
- Role-play the conversation with a friend, change role and take on the person to whom you make the request.

Like most of the strategies in this book, assertiveness is a skill, and therefore you will get better at it with practice.

Seeking professional help

I encourage you to reach out for help. Overcoming an eating disorder is not easy, and having someone to support and help you is invaluable. Speak to your GP, or a member of your healthcare team, about a referral to a therapist. In addition to cognitive behavioural therapy, there are a number of different types of psychological treatment that can be used to treat eating disorders, such as cognitive analytic therapy (CAT), interpersonal therapy (IPT) and family therapy.

Advice for health professionals

Clinicians should maintain a high degree of attentiveness for the possibility of eating disorders amongst their patients, particularly when there is unexplained poor metabolic control and other signs listed in Box 6.2. A low threshold for referral to mental health professionals is warranted, as attention to eating problems may save lives amongst people with both diabetes and an eating disorder.

Box 6.2 Signs that may suggest the presence of an eating disorder (Criego, Crow, Goebel-Fabbri et al., 2009)

Overall deterioration in psychosocial functioning, including school attendance and performance, work functioning, and interpersonal relationships

Increasing neglect of diabetes management, including blood glucose monitoring, insulin titration and adherence to other medications

Erratic clinic attendance

Significant weight gain or loss

Frequent dieting and increased concern about meal planning and food composition

Poor body image or low self-esteem

Purging behaviours such as excessive exercise, laxative or diuretic use, or vomiting

Recurrent or frequent ketoacidosis

Bingeing

Depressive symptoms, including sad mood, low energy, poor concentration, fatigue, and disrupted sleep. Although depression and disturbed eating behaviour often coexist, poorly controlled diabetes can also directly contribute to depressive symptoms.

Many health professionals are fearful of 'teaching' eating disorder behaviours by mentioning them in routine clinic appointments. However, a stepped approach, using non-leading, open-ended questions such as the ones below, ensures that the topic can be approached with confidence.

How do you feel about your weight/shape/body?
Are you trying to lose weight at the moment?
Are you currently dieting?
Is it hard to control what you eat?
Do you ever adjust your insulin to control your weight?
Do you ever take less insulin than you should?

Of course, patients may not be ready to answer these kinds of questions truthfully, but the important thing is that you have started the conversation. You are conveying that you know about these issues and are open to talking about it.

One of the most important aspects of discussing eating issues is to establish a positive rapport with patients so that they know they are not going to be judged or subjected to unrealistic expectations. Because patients often feel ashamed of their struggle with eating issues, they need to learn to trust you as a healthcare professional, so that you can help them feel comfortable communicating openly and honestly about their difficulties. When trust, understanding and acceptance are established, patients may be more likely to engage in ongoing treatment (Goebel-Fabbri, 2009).

References

Colton, P., Rodin, G., Bergenstal, R. and Parkin, C. (2009). Eating disorders and diabetes: introduction and overview. *Diabetes Spectrum*, 22(3), 138–42.

Criego, A., Crow, S., Goebel-Fabbri, A. E., Kendall, D. and Parkin, C. (2009). Eating disorders and diabetes: screening and detection. *Diabetes Spectrum*, 22, 143–6.

Goebel-Fabbri, A. (2009). Disturbed eating behaviors and eating disorders in type 1 diabetes: clinical significance and treatment recommendations. *Current Diabetes Reports*, 9(2), 133–9.

Herpertz, S., Albus, C., Lichtblau, K., Köhle, K, Mann, K. and Senf, W. (2000) Relationship of weight and eating disorders in type 2 diabetic patients: a multicenter study. *International Journal of Eating Disorders* 28(1), 68–77.

Markowitz, J., Butler, D., Volkening, L., Antisdel, J. E., Anderson, B. and Laffel, L. (2010). Brief screening tool for disordered eating in diabetes: internal consistency and external validity in a contemporary sample of pediatric patients with type 1 diabetes. *Diabetes Care*, 33(3), 495–500.

Nielsen, S. (2002). Eating disorders in females with type 1 diabetes: an update of a meta-analysis. *European Eating Disorders Review*, 10(4), 241–54.

Schmidt, U. and Treasure, J. (2007) *Getting Better Bit(e) by Bit(e): A Survival Kit for Sufferers of Bulimia Nervosa and Binge Eating Disorder*. Routledge, Hove.

Further Reading and Resources

P. Cooper (2009). *Overcoming Bulimia Nervosa and Binge-Eating*. Robinson, London.

C. Freeman (2009). *Overcoming Anorexia Nervosa: A Self-Help Guide Using Cognitive Behavioural Techniques*. Robinson, London.

J. Gauntlett-Gilbert and C. Grace (2005). *Overcoming Weight Problems: A Self-Help Guide Using Cognitive Behavioural Techniques*. Robinson, London.

William Polonsky (1999). *Diabetes Burnout*. American Diabetes Association, Alexandria, VA.

U. Schmidt and J. Treasure (2007). *Getting Better Bit(e) by Bit(e): A Survival Kit for Sufferers of Bulimia Nervosa and Binge Eating Disorder*. Routledge, Hove.

Amy Stockwell Mercer (2012). *The Smart Woman's Guide to Diabetes*. Demos Health, New York.

Vieira, G. (2012). *Emotional Eating with Diabetes: Your Guide to Creating a Positive Relationship with Food*. Champlain College Publishing, Vermont.

Website

Diabetics With Eating Disorders: www.dwed.org.uk.

Beating Eating Disorders: http://www.b-eat.co.uk/

Behavioural Diabetes Institute: 'Eating Disorders and Diabetes' http://behavioraldiabetesinstitute.org/resources-diabetes-information-videos-BDI-lectures.html

7

Diabetes and Relationships

I am sure you have found that having diabetes does not just affect you in isolation. Dealing with the impact of diabetes on others around you, and managing the way that they relate to you and your diabetes, is an important set of skills to develop. This chapter will cover the three core areas of how diabetes affects the way you relate to others: with your healthcare team, in your family and social system, and in your sexual relationships.

Your Relationship with Healthcare Professionals

How can someone who only sees you once or twice a year for roughly 15 minutes at a time really 'get' what your experience of diabetes is like? Perhaps I am being a little controversial but I believe that, although you might expect them to, the diabetes doctor, nurse and dietician can't. But here's something you may not have thought of – they are not really there to.

Let me explain. Of course your healthcare team want you to be in control of your diabetes and be in good health. They are passionate about helping you to manage the delicate balance between food, medication and activity so that your blood glucose control is just right. This is fantastic: it is where their skills and expertise lie and they can give you advice based on their expert knowledge of the inner workings of the human body.

But, as committed and as dedicated as they are, they are not your psychologist, your counsellor or your friend. They aren't there to help you work on the *other* 'inner workings' of your body – your emotions.

Diabetes and Wellbeing: Managing the Psychological and Emotional Challenges of Diabetes Types 1 and 2, First Edition. Dr Jen Nash.
© 2013 John Wiley & Sons, Ltd. Published 2013 by John Wiley & Sons, Ltd.

That's why there can be a disconnect between your exectations and your experience of being heard in your diabetes appointments. It's thankfully becoming more and more recognized that managing diabetes takes an emotional toil as well as a physical one. Government health guidance is calling for greater access to psychological therapies, yet a recent survey in the UK showed that less than one third of diabetes centres have access to specialist psychological services (Diabetes UK, 2008). There are just not enough clinical psychologists to go around, unfortunately!

Potential challenges in the patient–healthcare professional relationship

Common experiences of encounters with healthcare professionals from the patient perspective are:

Feeling rushed
Being patronised, unintentionally or otherwise
Not being 'heard'
Feeling misunderstood
Not feeling free to talk about what is really of concern, for example that diabetes is getting you down
Feeling scolded or made to feel like a 'bad' patient
A pressure to lie about your blood glucose results or other health behaviour
Feeling that the healthcare professional is an 'expert' and can't be disagreed with
Not attending health appointments at all and avoiding healthcare professionals entirely.

Some common challenges from the healthcare professional's point of view are:

Not having as much time to spend with patients as they'd like
Feeling pressure to be the 'expert'
Feeling at a loss to know how to help
Working within an environment with scarce or stretched resources
Team conflict amongst colleagues
Working to meet government targets which prioritise 'hard' data such as the blood glucose levels of their patients over 'soft' data such as psychological wellbeing or quality of life

Realizing that they are not able to fully appreciate the lived experience of
   diabetes (being an 'expert' rather than an 'expert by experience')
Having to maintain the caring role at work when experiencing personal
   challenges in their life outside work.

How does it feel to read these two lists? Do any of them resonate with
your experience or surprise you? Just viewing the relationship from the
perspective of the 'other' can be helpful.

   Here are some tips for both the person with diabetes and the healthcare
professional.

For the person with diabetes: How to improve your relationship with your healthcare team

There are practical steps you can take today to feel more in control of this
relationship. Here are the three P's of improving your relationship with the
individuals in your healthcare team.

Plan   The first step is to plan for your appointment. Think back over the
last month: what has confused you, or surprised you, or encouraged you, or
frightened you about your diabetes? What are the three things you would
like to know or say to your health professional?

Participate   The second step is to be an active participant in your appointment. Polonsky (1999), suggests using the 'ABC' of effective communication
to aid you:

Assertiveness: express yourself with confidence
Brevity: speak as briefly as you can, keeping to the point at all times
Clarity: express yourself clearly, concisely and simply.

Often, writing down some bullet points before the appointment can be
helpful, covering the main topics of what you would like to talk about. You
can then choose to bring them to the appointment with you, or simply
have them in mind to recall them.

Partner   The third step is to understand and keep in mind that you and
the healthcare professional are equals. Rather than feeling like a passive
recipient of expertise, remember that you are two adults with an immense
wealth of expertise. The healthcare professional has expertise of diabetes

and the physical aspects of the condition; and you have extensive expertise gathered through your lived experience of daily life with diabetes. Together, you can share that expertise with one another to work towards the benefit of your health.

For some people reading this, this advice will seem quite straightforward and they will begin to implement these steps right away. For others, it can feel harder to make changes. This is when it can be helpful to think about what's going on for you emotionally that may be contributing to this resistance. To help you with this, you might like to try the following exercise.

Authority figures from your past

Think about your diabetes healthcare professional now. Conjure up an image of him or her in your mind.

Take notice of the feelings you are experiencing. Are they positive or negative?

Put a label on the feelings you are experiencing: contented, hopeless, angry, neutral, joyful, embarrassed, tense, supported, sad, uncertain, frightened, secure, shameful . . . ?

Now try to associate the feelings you have about the healthcare professional with the feelings you have about someone else in your life. Who from your past do you also have those kinds of feelings about?

What figure from your early life comes to mind? Your strict head teacher at school? A kindly babysitter? Your controlling parent? A supportive uncle?

This may seem like an odd exercise, and in some ways, it really is! But some models of psychological therapy (particularly psychodynamic models) offer the idea that the way we relate to people in our life today, particularly 'authority' figures such as healthcare professionals, are modelled on these early relationships.

Perhaps you relate to your diabetes doctor as if they were your controlling head teacher from school, who you always secretly wanted to rebel against. Or your supportive uncle, who if you smiled sweetly for long enough would always let you off the hook if you did something wrong. Seeing links with figures in your past can help you disentangle the ways you may be responding that are more relevant to your past, and instead interact with the professional as one adult with another.

Using CBT to Deal with Communicating with Health Professionals

Case study: Arjun

Arjun has been avoiding his appointments with the diabetes clinic. He has let his diet and exercise levels slip since he separated from his wife last year. He is certain his HbA1c is high; he has put on weight and he is not looking forward to going.

Step 1: What is the situation or event?

Thinking of an upcoming appointment.

Step 2: What do you tell yourself? What are the thoughts you notice running through your mind?

'I don't want to go.'
'My doctor does not understand me.'
'I don't want to be told off;'
'My results (HbA1c, weight, etc.) are going to be awful.'
'I'm a "bad" diabetic.'

Step 3: What is happening in your body and what do you do?

Mood – fearful, anxious
Body sensations – heart beating fast, shallow breathing, body tension
Behaviours – a desire to avoid, escape or cancel my appointment

Step 4: Challenge your thoughts by asking yourself some helpful questions

What is the evidence for and against this thought?
Is thinking this way helping me?
Are there other ways of thinking about this situation?
If a friend told me they were thinking this way, how would I respond?
Am I thinking in 'all or nothing' terms?
What other points of view are there?
How would someone else think about this?
How else could I think about it?
How would I think about this if I were feeling better?

What are the facts of the case?
How can I find out which way of thinking fits the facts best?
What is the evidence?
Could I be making a mistake in the way I am thinking?
Am I thinking straight?
Am I pressurizing myself?
Am I using the language of the extremist?
What is the worst thing that could happen?

Step 5: Come up with an alternative, balanced thought

'I don't want to go.' I don't want to go, but if I do go I will feel proud of myself and feel I've achieved something difficult/overcome a challenge.

There are many things in life that I've done which I didn't want to (e.g. go to a job interview, end a relationship that wasn't working, have a difficult conversation with someone), but I did it because I knew that the long-term result I wanted was worth the short-term pain. I can apply the same rationale to my health appointments: by being able to tolerate the difficult feelings I will have more personal control and power.

'My doctor does not understand me.' Although she does not seem to understand me, she does work with people with diabetes every single day. I can tell her I don't feel understood.

'I don't want to be told off.' If I feel I'm being told off, I can tell my doctor that that's how I feel. I can tell her that I've been reading this book and am trying to change the way I relate to my diabetes.

'My results (HbA1c, weight, etc.) are going to be awful.' If my results are disappointing, I will ask for my doctor/nurse's advice on how to set an achievable goal that I can aim to meet for my next appointment.

'I'm a "bad" diabetic.' Although I have a sense that I'm 'bad', this is just a thought or feeling, it's not a fact. I am not a bad person for not always prioritizing my diabetes health. I know I am a good person as [I helped my friend out, gave time or money to a charity, compromised so someone I care about could be happy]. Just as I wouldn't think that person with cancer who was scared to go to their appointments is 'bad', I'm not bad. There is a distinction between a less than good behaviour and my whole identity being bad.

Going to the doctor's after a long time away is a bit like exercising: at first it will be painful, but as the muscles get used and stronger, it will become easier, perhaps even enjoyable! (Or maybe not!) I need to exercise my health appointments muscle.

I will reward myself once I've been to the appointment: every time I think of it I will remind myself of the reward I will enjoy afterwards and how nice it will feel to engage in it. (Ideas are: buy a magazine, enjoy my favourite drink at my favourite coffee shop, meet up with a friend, engage in a favourite hobby, listen to some great music, watch a film, go for a relaxing walk in an appealing environment, read a book, organize a treat (a ticket to a sporting event, a trip to the cinema, a picnic, a day out with the family.)

Advice for the healthcare professional

'She says she wants to change but she always comes back and nothing is different.'

'Am I doing something wrong? No one seems to take any notice of my advice.'

'I always run out of time.'

'I'm stuck.'

'Some patients just make me feel like I'm rubbish at my job.'

'Why won't he do what he needs to do to care for his health?.'

Have you ever had thoughts like these? You are not alone. Many clinicians struggle to feel they are good enough. The section that follows aims to help you think about your patients' actions from a different perspective and introduces some strategies to help you.

The patient is doing what is right for them   You might not 'get' why your patient is not caring well for their health. People act in accordance with their feelings, beliefs, cultural norms and values, and your belief systems may be very different to your patient's. Exploring the background to your patient's beliefs can give you both clarity. Behaviour that is difficult for you to understand usually stems from a person's belief about its value, or is based in habits that might be difficult to alter. By asking questions in an open, enquiring way, you will get an insight into the beliefs that are driving their behaviours and actions.

How to improve your relationship with your patient

Set an agenda   Time in a consultation is short, and you will both have an agenda to fulfil. It is good practice to set the frame of the space. For example:

'We have 15 minutes together today [*point towards or indicate the clock*]. I will be keeping an eye on the time for us. Let's prioritize how we are going to spend this time so we use it wisely. What would you most like to discuss?'

Make a note of their answers. If the client starts going off at length, you could say, 'Can I pause you for a moment? For now I just want to get the main areas and then we can focus on each in turn. To recap, we've got [insert agenda items]. I would like to add one in too, which is [share agenda item]. We may not have time to cover them all today, in which case I will keep a note and add them to the agenda for next time. So we can prioritize, which is the most important item to cover today?'

Keep track of time. When you notice you are in the final five minutes, let the client know. 'We've got five minutes left so let's make a plan to guide you between now and the next time we meet.'

Help the client become active   Invite the client to be active within the session. You could give them a sheet of paper and a pen (and a surface to write on). Do be sensitive if they are not keen to write, or their literacy levels are low.

Empathy   Empathize, empathize, empathize. Research into the efficacy of various forms of psychological therapy demonstrates that the most important factor in any successful therapy intervention is the relationship. How are relationships developed? Through shared experience, being listened to and accepted. Give permission for your patient to find things difficult.

Focus on the issue that the patient is concerned about   Often the patient will be most concerned about something completely unrelated to their diabetes: financial worries, or a sick relative or a relationship breakdown. You do not have to be an expert in this or have a solution to it; simply acknowledging it and helping the person identify how to gain their own solution or move forward can be very helpful.

Be curious about successes   Be curious about any movement at all in a positive direction. Ask your patient, 'What is going well with your diabetes?' (If they reply 'nothing' you can always let them know that coming to the appointment is a positive step!) 'What was different on these days? What helped and what got in the way?' Have a look at Chapter 9 for more about focusing on successes.

Keep the goals very small   Goals need to be small, the smaller the better in fact. Success builds on success. Yes, your client may need to lose three stone in weight. But being thoughtful about how to cut out the biscuit with the cup of tea is an important step towards an overall goal (the extra 100 or more calories, a few times a day, over a year, really adds up!). Do encourage and praise your patient, and notice times when they may be quick to discount their success. Bring it out into the open and congratulate them for these with a simple, 'Well done'. Be ready to encourage and praise.

Normalize   Let your patient know that they are not unusual. Tell them that you have worked with lots of other people who have struggled with similar issues. Reassure them that their experience is 'normal'.

Problem-solve in the context of everyday life   Behaviour change can be theory-driven, but it also needs to fit into everyday life. Think flexibly about how a goal might be implemented and the unspoken barriers that are really preventing change from being realized. Ask your client, 'What might get in the way of implementing this change?' Problem-solve with them. For example:

Do they forget to test their blood glucose? Could they move their kit somewhere they will see it often, such as by the phone or on the kitchen counter?

Will they need to ask their partner to take on childcare responsibilities to allow them to do some exercise a few times a week? When and how will they do this?

Look out for systemic issues that are obstacles to behaviour change. In the example above, is the real problem that they do not have the skills to ask their partner for support? In that case a valuable conversation could be had about how to equip the client with the communication skills they need to convey to their partner the importance of giving support.

As diabetes is woven so intricately into a person's life, personal goals that are not obviously about their condition are still valid. They are likely also to have implications for health at some stage.

Be comfortable with being silent   In 'real' life we usually have to feel comfortable with someone before we can be comfortable with being silent with them. A healthcare appointment is not 'real' life; of course it is based in reality but it is not subject to the same customs as everyday interactions. Healthcare professionals can feel a pressure to fill the gaps, to provide more information, to squeeze much into a short period of time. Avoid this. The diabetes consultation may be the one time the patient actually thinks about their diabetes, and silence can be an important part of cognitive processing. If you struggle with silence, count backwards in your head or think of the words of a song to help you. If the silence goes on for so long that you think it is because they don't know where to start, simply reflecting this can be beneficial: 'It's difficult to know where to start' or 'It's hard to know what to say'.

Finish with next steps   Many patients report struggling to recall the advice provided to them in consultations. Counter this by recapping what you have spoken about and the strategies you have suggested. Invite the patient to write these down to aid their memory.

What is my personal goal from today?
What will I do to achieve this goal?
Weekly review: How am I doing towards goal achievement?

Go easy on yourself: you are not responsible   As a healthcare professional you will want to do the best for your patients. However, you are not their parent, and it is not your job to 'solve' their health problems. They are adults and they are ultimately responsible for their health decisions. You are a partnership, and for a partnership to work, collaboration is crucial.

Anderson and Funnell (2005) remind us that as much of 98 per cent of diabetes care is carried out by the individual with diabetes themselves. The patient's health and wellbeing are therefore a product of their self-management decisions during the routine action of their everyday life. Healthcare professionals are responsible for doing all they can to ensure their patients are making informed self-management decisions, but they are not responsible for the carrying out of these decisions.

Keep a list of discussion questions nearby   If you are changing your style in the way suggested here, it is likely to be a while before you feel completely natural using it. It may be helpful to have some questions prepared in advance. Here are some suggestions.

How are you?
What are you struggling with at the moment?
How could you change that?
What would help you?
How have you made changes in the past?
How would you feel if you were able to achieve that?
What was that like?
How did that feel?
What frustrates you most about your diabetes?
What do you think about your results?
Tell me what you have been thinking about in relation to your diabetes?
Can you describe how your diabetes affects your day-to-day life?
Which aspects of your condition would you most like us to talk about today?

Be aware of power   Historically, the healthcare system has been one of the clinician as expert and the patient as recipient of expertise: you study and train for many years and then impart this knowledge to your patient in the context of the consultation. This model works well for acute care settings, but for a condition like diabetes, in which most of the care is done by the patient outside the healthcare setting, it obviously has limitations. Educating your patient that they are an 'expert by experience' and have the true power is an important step.

The part you can control is the process: the questions you ask and the way that you ask them, the way you respond to your patient, the way you help them to be thoughtful about their health. Improve these and you are doing well. If in doubt:

Remain curious and simply ask questions about the person's experience.
Experiment with not giving any advice at all, unless directly asked for it.

CBT for the Healthcare Professional

This book has offered CBT strategies to tackle the emotional impact of diabetes. But being a helping professional is emotionally demanding and there is no shame in feeling a bit burned out yourself occasionally. You might like to look at the advice in Chapter 4 about being kind to yourself and ensuring you have a fair balance of duties and pleasure in your life.

Case study: Shahaam

Shahaam is a Diabetes Specialist Nurse who enjoys her work but sometimes feels overwhelmed when working with patients who are in distress. She is quick to feel inadequate and criticizes herself when consultations do not go as well as he would like.

Step 1: What is the situation or event?

Before an appointment with a patient whose consultation did not go well last time.

Step 2: What do you tell yourself? What are the thoughts you notice running through your mind?

'I'm no good.'
'I've failed.'
'I'm stuck.'
'I feel like a rubbish nurse.'

Step 3: What is happening in your body and what do you do?

Mood – fearful, anxious
Body sensations – heart beating fast, shallow breathing, body tension
Behaviours – a desire to avoid or escape the appointment

Step 4: Challenge your thoughts by asking yourself some helpful questions

What is the evidence for and against this thought?
Is thinking this way helping me?
Are there other ways of thinking about this situation?
If a friend told me they were thinking this way, how would I respond?

Am I thinking in 'all or nothing' terms?
What other points of view are there?
How would someone else think about this?
How else could I think about it?
How would I think about this if I were feeling better?
What are the facts of the case?
How can I find out which way of thinking fits the facts best?
What is the evidence?
Could I be making a mistake in the way I am thinking?
Am I thinking straight?
Am I pressurizing myself?
Am I using the language of the extremist?
What is the worst thing that could happen?

Step 5: Come up with an alternative, balanced thought

'I'm no good.' I am going to try something new by asking some more open questions. That way, I will feel proud of myself for achieving something.

'I've failed.' Simply offering this person a space to think about their diabetes, and asking them questions (no matter how much they might want answers), is my way of giving value to this person.

'I'm stuck.' I probably feel stuck because the patient is stuck too. I could share that I feel stuck with her. Naming it and sharing the dilemma might help, paradoxically. Some patients are at different readiness for change.

'I feel like a rubbish nurse.' Although I sometimes feel rubbish, that does not mean I *am* rubbish. I have received good feedback from other patients and colleagues who have worked with me. Just like I do not get on with every single person I meet in my personal life, my style will not be the perfect fit for every patient. It doesn't make me rubbish.

Relationships in Your Family and Social System

Diabetes does not just affect you; it has the potential to impact each of your close relationships too, with your spouse or partner and those in your wider family network. Have you ever thought about how those around you help or hinder your diabetes care?

Diabetes can of course cause worry and anxiety for the person with diabetes; but the irony is it often causes even more concern in those around them. This is often because, while the person with diabetes is busily occupied engaging in their diabetes self-care, doing something and therefore getting a sense of control over their health, those alongside them may be feeling there is little they can actually do to help, and therefore have may use other, less direct ways to gain control of their anxiety.

This anxiety can express itself in a variety of quite contrasting ways. The two most common are feeling isolated and/or unsupported by those close to you, and the opposite: feeling blamed or hassled by your family. But have you considered that it may be anxiety that is causing them to react in these potentially unhelpful ways?

Do you recognize your situation in any of the following scenarios?

Perhaps they criticize you for being overweight, or reprimand you for not keeping good blood glucose control, which can feel very blaming.

Or maybe your loved ones completely ignore your diabetes, leaving you feeling alone and isolated without support.

Perhaps they seem to tell everyone you meet that 'He/she's diabetic, they can't eat that', drawing everyone's attention to the ways in which you are 'different', when all you want to do is blend in like everyone else.

You may feel that those close to you are observing you at every turn, checking what you are eating and how much attention you are paying to your medication and exercise regimes.

Maybe they seem to feel the need to 'advise' you at all times, which can feel more like lecturing than helpful suggestions.

Whatever way diabetes is affecting your close relationships, here are my top tips to help you manage better.

Communicate

The first step in making a positive change in a relationship is to have an honest and straightforward conversation with your loved one. In many situations in which diabetes is causing a strain on a relationship, the problem does not get talked about openly. When conflicts are buried in this way, arguments and resentments can be expressed in other ways, with the true source of the conflict unacknowledged.

Try and plan what you would like to say beforehand so it comes across as
   calmly as possible.
State what you are unhappy with in a matter-of-fact way.
Make clear that you realize they love you and are trying to help, but there
   might be more useful ways they can do so if you think about it together.
Sandwich the potential criticism between two pieces of praise. For example,
   'I know you really care about me and I am grateful for the way you
   help me. When you ... [describe what they say or do], 'it makes me
   feel ... [insert emotion – upset, guilty, embarrassed, etc.]'. I know that
   you are trying to support me and want to find a way we can work together
   to make things better.'

Ask for help

Be clear about what is the best form of help your loved one could give
you. For example, perhaps they are criticizing you for your need to lose
weight, when it would be more helpful if you could learn how to prepare
healthy meals together. Or maybe they are nagging at you to test your blood
glucose more, when what would really be helpful would be if they praised
and encouraged you with a smile and a hug when they did notice you test.

Take personal responsibility

Are you being honest with yourself and taking personal responsibility for
your diabetes self-care? Often those around you may see that you are
'sticking your head in the sand' about your diabetes care and may feel at a
loss to know what to do to help. Nagging or hassling you may be the only
way they can try to relate to you about the problems they see. Perhaps you
always say 'I'm fine' when asked about your diabetes, even if it is evident
that all is not fine. Out of love and worry the person close to you wants to
help you to change. By being honest with yourself and those around you
about what you are struggling with, you can begin to take steps together
to improve your diabetes health, avoiding the need for your loved one to
resort to unhelpful pestering behaviour.

Seek professional help

If you have implemented the steps above and are still struggling, think about
seeking professional help. Often, having a third, emotionally uninvolved
person to listen and help you problem-solve can really help you move

forward together productively. It may be challenging for one or both or you to keep calm or to see the other's point of view when talking about diabetes, so seeing a family therapist or counsellor can really help you have useful conversations. Just one session can be helpful in getting you unstuck. Resources are recommended at the end of this chapter.

Using CBT to Help Manage Relationships

Case study: Derek

Derek has been feeling unsupported by his partner Maria ever since he got diagnosed. He knows there can be times when he is not as worried about his health as she is, but he does not want to be constantly reminded of his diabetes, which she seems to feel the need to do.

Step 1: What is the situation or event?

Being criticized by Maria, talking about my diabetes with everyone at the party.

Step 2: What do you tell yourself? What are the thoughts you notice running through your mind?

'Why is she acting like this?'
'She doesn't care about me.'
'This is so annoying.'
'I wish she'd shut up.'
'She makes me feel like a failure.'

Step 3: What is happening in your body and what do you do?

Mood – angry, short-tempered, anxious, frustrated
Body sensations – heart beating fast, shallow breathing
Behaviours – leave the room, fuming, and then snap at her later about something completely unrelated

Step 4: Challenge your thoughts by asking yourself some helpful questions

What is the evidence for and against this thought?
Is thinking this way helping me?

Are there other ways of thinking about this situation?

If a friend told me they were thinking this way, how would I respond?

Am I thinking in 'all or nothing' terms?

What other points of view are there?

How would someone else think about this?

How else could I think about it?

How would I think about this if I were feeling better?

What are the facts of the case?

How can I find out which way of thinking fits the facts best?

What is the evidence?

Could I be making a mistake in the way I am thinking?

Am I thinking straight?

Am I pressurizing myself?

Am I using the language of the extremist?

What is the worst thing that could happen?

Step 5: Come up with an alternative, balanced thought

'Why is she acting like this?' I know Maria does love me; she has shown me she does by [insert your own example here].

'She doesn't care about me.' She does care about me; I'm just annoyed at her. I'm going to discuss how I feel with her.

'This is so annoying.' I'm going to ask Maria tomorrow if she can try not to mention my diabetes to others unless I do first.

'I wish she'd shut up.' I have a right to feel this way, but I need to chat to her about it at a time when we are both calm.

'She makes me feel like a failure.' I'm going to direct her to the ways that she can help me.

By implementing these steps, you will improve your most important relationships – with your diabetes and with your loved ones.

Sexual Difficulties

Encountering problems with sexual response is a common experience for both men and women with diabetes. Not only can diabetes affect your physical functioning, there can also be psychological factors that interfere with a full and rewarding sex life. Problems with sexual function can be very distressing, and affect the quality of your life as well as your relationships. Although help is available, many people (both with and without diabetes) find sexual difficulties an embarrassing topic to talk about in the context of a health appointment, and therefore refrain from being open with their doctor or nurse about their difficulties. This section will help you to become more familiar with the different ways your sexual responses may be affected, give you strategies to help you tackle the psychological difficulties that might be getting in your way, and empower you to talk to your doctor or nurse about how they can help you. The section is written, for simplicity, in terms of a heterosexual relationship, but can be adapted to same-sex relationships.

Male sexual problems

Erectile dysfunction (also known as impotence) means that you are not able to obtain or keep an erection long enough for sexual intercourse. An erection is caused by the flow of blood into the penis and the blocking of the small blood vessels, making the penis hard. In some studies more than 50% of males with diabetes admitted difficulties with sexual function, rising to more than 75% for men over the age of 70. To put this into context, about 1 in 10 men over 40 years old have erectile dysfunction whether they have diabetes or not. Many factors along with diabetes can contribute to difficulties with sexual response. These include:

Drinking alcohol
Smoking
Taking non-prescription drugs
Medications such as certain antidepressants
Injury to the penis
Damage to the spinal cord
Nerve damage caused by operations to the bladder, bowel or prostate gland
Poor blood supply to the penis due to blockage of the artery caused by peripheral arterial disease
Producing less testosterone than your body needs
High blood pressure.

Female sexual problems

Women with diabetes are also at risk from difficulties with sexual response, and although these are not as visually obvious as for men, they are just as upsetting and difficult to contend with.

Physical problems are:

Dry vagina caused by high blood glucose levels
Greater proneness to yeast infections, making sexual intercourse uncomfortable
Loss of skin sensation around the vagina area, reducing the pleasure experienced.

In addition to physical explanations for sexual difficulties, there are also emotional reasons why you may be encountering problems relating sexually to your partner. These affect both men and women. Some of these are:

Stress
Depression and low mood
Anxiety and worry
Conflict with your partner
Issues regarding how sex is viewed in your religion or culture
Homosexuality
Bereavement
Illness or ill health
Being in an accident
Previous abuse
Infertility
Disability

Gain support for the physical side of sex

The first step is to have a physical examination by your GP or healthcare team and take advantage of medical treatments or aids that they recommend to you. For men with diabetes, Viagra and similar prescription medications can be incredibly helpful and they have no adverse impact on diabetes control. Do not buy any medicines to treat erectile dysfunction over the internet. It may seem appealing as you can get help anonymously without having to approach a potentially embarrassing topic at clinic, but there is no guarantee that what you are buying is genuine. It is also important that your healthcare team are aware of all the medications you are taking.

Other general guidelines for improving sexual response for both men and women are:

Weight loss, smoking cessation and cutting down on alcohol intake

Improving glucose control or changing some of your medicines. If the sexual difficulty coincided with a sudden worsening of your glucose control or with starting a different drug, it is important to look at these factors

Testosterone replacement therapy: a blood test may indicate low testosterone levels which can be corrected with testosterone replacement therapy.

It is natural to feel embarrassment about discussing sexual problems with healthcare professionals. Remember they have heard similar problems before and will not be fazed by them. Indeed, they will respect that you are able to be open about it and seek help. Remember the first line will be the most challenging; once that is done the clinician will steer the conversation for you. Some ideas for conversation starters are listed below.

I'm having problems in bed.
I'm struggling with sex/my sex life.
My [penis, 'equipment', etc.] isn't working as it should.
I've got something I'm a bit embarrassed to mention .... (The clinician may pre-empt what you are about to say.)
I was hoping that you might be able to help me with this problem I am having.
I think I've got ED/erectile dysfunction.
I can't get a hard-on.

How to manage the emotional impact of sexual difficulties

If you have been checked out by your healthcare team and there are no obvious physical problems, then shifting focus to psychological strategies can be helpful.

Enjoyment of sex goes beyond the act of intercourse that culminates in an orgasm. Enjoyment of the sexual experience involves a whole range of factors, including your past experiences of sex, your appearance, your confidence physically and sexually and so on. Early traumatic experiences involving sex and negative beliefs about sex inherited from family values and attitudes can hinder the sexual experience. The sensate exercises here can help overcome these and increase your confidence in your own body. Remember that knowing what turns you on is crucial to helping a partner to learn what your tastes are.

A plan for tackling sexual difficulties: sensate focus
(adapted from Ford, 2005)

The aim of sensate focus is to learn new ways to be intimate together, that do not focus on erection or orgasm. It is designed as the starting point for all sexual problems (for men and women). It allows you to get out of the trap of the topic of sex feeling conflictual, and helps you renew your enjoyment in your own and each other's bodies. This takes the pressure off in the short term, providing a good foundation for better relating. The whole exercise is planned to take five weeks, although it may take longer if you need to allow more time for particular stages. In the first week, you need to plan and find time for three sessions, each lasting approximately 1–2 hours. For best results, it is advisable to agree with each other not to have sex or masturbate outside of these sessions.

Week 1   You take it in turns to be the 'active partner'; so decide who will go first.

The passive partner lies down on their tummy on the bed, getting as relaxed and comfortable as possible.

The exercise is designed to be done in silence so only comment if something is uncomfortable or painful. Remaining quiet helps to avoid embarrassment and also aids your concentration.

If one or both of you feel embarrassed being naked (perhaps because it has been a while, or because of weight gain or a scar following an operation) then you can begin wearing underwear or a towel. These can be removed in future sessions as you get more comfortable.

Active partner, it is your role to give a massage, but a slightly different massage to the ones you may have given in the past. This one uses more of your senses: sight, sound, smell, taste and touch.

Start by touching the top of your partner's head. Feel the shape and size, smell the head and hair, run your fingers through the hair, use soft massage strokes all around the head and neck.

Move down to the shoulder, kneading, squeezing, using whatever strokes you like. Massage the back, run your fingers down the spine, kiss, taste, pummel the skin, for women you can use your breasts or hair if it is long enough – whatever feels good.

Next move on to the buttocks, again using whatever stroke feels good. Work down the tops of the legs over the calves and down towards the feet and toes. Firm hand movements are better than soft fluttery ones which may be ticklish.

Spend about 15 minutes doing this exercise, and then tweak your partner's big toe to indicate that it is time for them to turn over so they are lying on their back.

Start again from the top, exploring the face, nose and lips, kissing, gently licking, tasting and touching. Move on to the chest but avoid breasts and nipples as they are off limits for now. Massage the chest and tummy, then the arms and hands. Lick, gently bite and suck the fingers.

Do not touch the vulva or penis at this stage. Massage the tops of the legs, work down over the knees and shins to the top of the feet. This should take another 15 minutes, making half an hour in total.

When you have finished, it is time to swap places; the passive partner becomes active and follows the same routine as you did. When you are done, put on a towel or robe, cuddle up and talk to one another about the experience and your feelings.

Sensate focus: questions to ask each other

What felt good?

What did you enjoy?

Were there any difficult parts?

What have you learned for yourself?

Which role felt more comfortable?

Did you feel any pressure in either role?

Did you feel anxious at all? If so did the anxiety lessen or increase as the exercise progressed?

Week 2   Week 2 follows the same pattern as week 1, but incorporates experimenting with lotions, talk, creams, massage oils, food or drink.

Think about smell. What smells do you like? What feels good? What looks good? It is important that when you are the active partner you use the products you like rather than what your partner likes. You can always wash it off afterwards. Have some fun and be imaginative. Try feathers, chocolate, silky material. Do be careful if you have a skin complaint or allergy.

You can give feedback (such as 'that's nice' or 'softer/harder') but keep talk to a minimum.

The sexual areas are still off limits during this week.

Again, attempt to complete three sessions over the week, talking over and recording your findings after each one and, if you need to, taking time for one or two additional session so that you are completely comfortable before moving on to week three.

Week 3 The following week, repeat again everything you have done but now include the breasts and genital areas.

Do not pay any particular attention to the sexual areas, but as you make your journey over your partner's body give them as much attention as you would any other part of the body.
The focus is on building trust and confidence.
Talk about each session afterwards in the same way as previously, and only move on when you feel ready to.

Week 4 Week 4 is about learning what each of you enjoys.

Having completed the massage as before, focus on the sexual areas.
Take a look at your partner's penis/vulva. Note the colour and texture of the skin, feel the warmth, feel her breasts and his nipples, note the size and colour. Do no more than simply look and gently touch.
Should you start to feel any anxiety, stop and talk to teach other about what is making you feel uncomfortable. As with any of the stages described above, do not move on to the next stage until you feel OK. Once the exercise is complete, discuss it together in the usual way.

Week 5 Week five is about giving and receiving pleasure for mutual enjoyment.

Repeat all of the steps in week four above, but now tell each other what feels good as it happens.
Provide feedback about what you are enjoying: 'that's nice', or 'more of that', or 'softer/harder', etc.

At this point, the programmes change depending on whether you are struggling with erectile dysfunction or orgasmic dysfunction.

Next steps for erectile dysfunction

Week 6

Think about how you can pleasure your partner. Some men prefer to give pleasure first, particularly if their desire drops after they have had an orgasm. If you both know in advance the order you are going to do things, it helps the flow of the session.

If you are a bit uncomfortable with body fluids following ejaculation then you may also want to have a box of tissues nearby.

Lie down on the bed with your head at the foot end. Your partner needs to sit between your legs with her back supported by pillows against the bed-head.

Put your legs over hers (you may need to bend them) in the kind of position you might adopt to row a boat. You will need to move your bottom up the bed slightly so that your partner can comfortably sit and hold your penis. If your partner is unable to sit this way you may need to experiment with other ways that are comfortable, yet give easy access to your penis.

Your partner needs to stimulate your penis in a way that feels good to you. To start with, try stimulating yourself with your partner's hand on yours so that she can feel exactly how you like to be touched. Enjoy the sensations this produces.

When she has got the right movement, swap over so that she holds your penis and you put your hand over hers until you feel she has got the pressure, rhythm and speed just right.

Your partner continues to stimulate you by herself. You may need to repeat this a few times in order to get it completely right. Use fantasy if you find this helpful.

Questions for discussion

How did this feel?
Did you enjoy the experience?
Were you able to get a good erection using the exercise?
Did you feel anxious at all?
Did your penis fail to respond?
Were you able to use fantasy to help?

Feedback, now and in the later stages, is essential. You and your partner need to share thoughts and feelings about what happens in the session in order to learn from the experience. Repeat this exercise two or three times (more if you like) until your erection is good and firm.

Week 7

Prepare as before.

When ready, move into the 'rowing boat' position and get your partner to stimulate you to a good erection in the way she knows how.

When you are fully erect she is to stop stimulating you. Let the erection go down.

Next, she is to repeat the process, stimulating you to full erection and then stopping to allow the erection to go down again.

Repeat this a third time.

On the fourth occasion, she will stimulate you to a full erection again, but this time you are free to ejaculate if you can.

Discuss together what happened and learn from the experience.

Questions for discussion

How did you feel?

Did you manage one erection, two erections, or three?

If you ejaculated, did you enjoy it?

Were you in touch with and focusing on the sensations in your genitals?

Did you feel anxious at all?

Did your partner feel anxious?

Repeat the whole exercise again two or three times (or more) until you are able to get a good erection three times in the session, ejaculating on the final time. Move on only when you are completely comfortable with this week.

Week 8

Prepare in the usual way.

This time your partner positions herself on top of you, sitting on the tops of your legs.

Taking hold of your penis, she should stimulate you to a full erection and then let it go down as before. You may need to stimulate your partner to ensure she is aroused enough for the next step, or use some additional lubricant.

This time when she restimulates you to a full erection, she can put your
   penis inside her. She only needs to move enough to keep the erection for
   a short while.
When ready, she comes off your penis and stimulates you to orgasm.

Questions for discussion

How did you get on?
Did you have a good enough erection for her to put your penis inside her
   vagina?
How did that feel?
If you found you lost your erection as she tried to insert it, she needs to
   restimulate your penis and try again.
Did your penis not get erect due to anxiety?
If so, think about what made you anxious. This will help you avoid anxiety
   next time.
Did you think about fantasy?
Were you concentrating and enjoying yourself?

Discuss together what each of you observed and learned from the exercise.
Give her lots of cuddles and hugs for being there for you. Repeat two or
three more times (or more) until you have successfully managed the whole
of week 8.

Week 9

Repeat all of week 8.
This time, if you would like to thrust then do so.
If you feel good about how things are going, ejaculate inside her vagina.

Questions for discussion

How did that feel?
Were you able to thrust and keep your erection?
Better still, did you ejaculate?

If the answer is yes, repeat the exercise two or three times (or more)
to consolidate what you have achieved and to build up pleasurable
experiences.
   If you lost your erection at any point during the process, go back to being
stimulated outside the vagina a few times, and then move on to putting
your penis inside again. Repeat the exercise until all of week 9 is completed.

Week 10   Now your erection is reliable, try experimenting with different positions. Have fun!

If your partner becomes dry during the exercises (it's hard to stay fully aroused for long periods) you might like to apply a lubricant to help with insertion. You can use it directly on the penis or vagina, or both.

If you have found the above programme difficult to complete, you may need to think about why that was. Do you feel exposed? Do you still think you are going to fail? Talk to your partner about your concerns. She can't help you if you don't share what is going on. Do you think negatively about your body? Go to the section on CBT below and use the exercises to help you.

Next steps for orgasmic dysfunction in women: body awareness exercise

Having difficulty experiencing an orgasm can cause a lot of upset for women and put strain on a relationship. Just as with male sexual problems, having problems reaching orgasm is often accompanied by lots of pressure to succeed, both from the woman and from a partner who may well be questioning his ability as a lover. Childhood messages relating to sex and intimacy can leave an unhelpful legacy causing a lack of freedom to feel sexually attractive and experiencing guilt or shame about your body or feeling sexy. Masturbation can also be a taboo subject and some women feel unable to try it. The problem is sometimes also connected to a fear of letting go (or 'surrendering' to a man) or of being out of control. Anxiety can build up and culminate in questions like, 'Do I look foolish?' or worse, 'I take so long; is he getting bored?' For older women in particular, stress incontinence (leaking of urine from the bladder at orgasm) can be an issue, which also can be very inhibiting.

Whatever the reason, the programme outlined here is designed to help you overcome inhibitions, reduce tension and anxiety and help you take control of your own body.

Week 6

Make sure you are nice and relaxed before you begin.
Prepare and work through week 5 until you are both feeling aroused and turned on. Discuss when your partner would like his orgasm.

Ask your partner to sit propped up against some pillows or cushions, sit between his legs with your back to him and lie back against his chest.

Pull his arms around you until you both feel relaxed in this position. When you are ready, your partner can begin to caress and stroke you.

Using your hand, gently stimulate your clitoris until your body is responding by opening up (arousal phase).

Turn yourself on by concentrating your mind on the pleasure you are experiencing, or focus on a fantasy.

Ask your partner to put his hand over yours so that he can feel how you like to be touched. Let him feel the pressure, speed and motion that gives you pleasure.

When you are ready, let him try your technique himself. Give him lots of encouragement and feedback on what is good.

If he does not get it quite right, put your hand on top of his and guide him gently. Let him try again on his own until you are happy with the result. Then let your orgasm come and enjoy it.

How did that feel? Did you both enjoy it . . . or did your partner find it hard to get the technique right? Do not worry, it is bound to feel a little strange to start with. Practice and familiarity will help overcome these feelings. The important thing is that you are open and honest with each other. If you have ever pretended to have orgasms in the past, avoid any urge you may now have to pretend that everything is working fine when it is not. Repeat the exercise two or three times, or as many as you need in order to feel comfortable with each other. Additional lubrication can help if it takes a while to get to orgasm.

Week 7

Repeat stage 1 to arousal.

When you are both ready, ask your partner to lie down, and sit across the tops of his legs so that you can arouse each other easily

Use additional lubrication on his penis if you wish. Sit up and put his penis inside your vagina and slowly lower yourself onto him (use cushions under your knees if you need extra height)

You or your partner can stimulate your clitoris at the same time as you gently move up and down on his penis.

Use orgasmic triggers: hold your head back, arch your back, tense your muscles. Increase speed to increase stimulation.

This position is excellent for achieving orgasm. Move yourself around to maximize sensation and pleasure, continue until you feel your vaginal muscles start to tighten, and then allow your orgasm to come.

You may like to stimulate your partner to orgasm now if you haven't already done so.

How did that feel? Were you able to orgasm? If not, don't worry, as you were probably very close. As long as you focus and don't allow yourself to become anxious or distracted, with practice it will happen. Repeat this exercise two or three times or more – as many as you like. Have fun learning how to make your body respond. Encourage your partner to tell you how he feels.

Week 8

Experiment with different positions and different ways to stimulate your clitoris. Your partner can begin thrusting as well.

If you have not been orgasmic during penetration, discuss how and when you would like to be stimulated to orgasm.

Many women do not experience orgasm through penetration alone. If that is the case, you can experiment with enjoying an orgasm using a vibrator, or orally. Repeat this exercise two or three times (or more) until you are regularly enjoying your sexual relationship together.

If you have experienced any problems during the programme, there are other things you can try. If you have never masturbated, you may find it helpful to get used to enjoying your body in this way and learn what you need to do to allow your body to respond. Once you are orgasmic on your own you can share the information gained with your partner and then work through the above programme again. As with many skills, it will take trial and error, patience, and help and support from your partner to overcome your sexual difficulty. Remember, do not put yourself under pressure, go at your own pace and you will get there in the end.

Other aspects of sexual relationships

In addition to working specifically on the sexual aspects of your relationship, it is important to attend to its other elements.

Communication The sexual programme above will help with communication. Allow time each day to really communicate with one another. Even 10 minutes a day is a great start. Really listen to what your partner is saying.

Empathize with what they are saying. Attend to their body language and do not offer solutions or try to problem-solve unless explicitly asked to.

Express conflict   Hurts and conflicts that are unvoiced are toxic to a relationship. A mirroring can occur, in which conflict isn't expressed openly, and so sexual love isn't expressed in the bedroom.

Set goals of spending romantic time together   Life is really busy, and it can be difficult to fit in quality time to relate with each other. It is therefore important to make a specific date to do this. Plan to have a relative or friend watch the children and decide what you would like to do: have a meal, go for a coffee, see a film, have a walk in the park, or even just stay at home with a DVD, but with no distractions and the phone turned off.

Other ways of giving love   We all give and receive love in a multitude of different ways and demonstrating our love is an important way of showing our feelings. Chapman (1992) has put forward an idea that we each have our own personal 'love language', one type of expression that is more dominant for us than the other ones.

Words of affirmation: receiving compliments, or hearing the words 'I love you'.

Quality time: enjoying your full, undivided attention makes this person feel very loved and special.

Receiving gifts: although few people would say they didn't enjoy receiving gifts, for this person it is the thoughtfulness and effort behind the gift which are prized.

Acts of service: being helped with the burden of responsibilities in small and big ways is important for this person.

Physical touch: while this can mean sexual touching, tender touching such as holding hands, hugs, pats and touches on the arm or face are also ways to show love.

Think with your partner about which ones you each particularly enjoy and be on the lookout for opportunities when you engage in each other's love language.

Raise your self-esteem   Sexual difficulties can knock the confidence of both men and women who are affected by them, so you may need to work on your self-esteem.

Keep a diary or record each day of three things you are proud of, have done well or like about yourself. For example, 'I had that difficult conversation with my colleague.'

Say something complimentary to yourself every time you look in a mirror: 'Your eyes look nice today', 'you have a delicate nose, ears, a good-shaped face, healthy hair, etc.', 'I feel good today', 'I did that really well'.

Using CBT to Deal with Sexual Difficulties

Case study: Robert

Robert has been struggling with erectile dysfunction for a few months now and although his partner, Francesca, is understanding and supportive, he still notices his mind wandering to negative thoughts about himself and his inability to pleasure her in bed.

Step 1: What is the situation or event?

Thinking back to a recent sexual experience with Francesca that did not go well.

Step 2: What do you tell yourself? What are the thoughts you notice running through your mind?

'I can't do this.'
'This is embarrassing.'
'It's not working as it should.'
'I'll never be normal.'
'Francesca will think I don't love her or fancy her any more.'

Step 3: What is happening in your body and what do you do?

Mood – fearful, anxious
Body sensations – heart beating fast, shallow breathing, flushed face due to embarrassment
Behaviours – want to avoid being close to Francesca, in case it leads somewhere

Step 4: Challenge your thoughts by asking yourself some helpful question:

What is the evidence for and against this thought?

Is thinking this way helping me?
Are there other ways of thinking about this situation?
If a friend told me they were thinking this way, how would I respond?
Am I thinking in 'all or nothing' terms?
What other points of view are there?
How would someone else think about this?
How else could I think about it?
How would I think about this if I were feeling better?
What are the facts of the case?
How can I find out which way of thinking fits the facts best?
What is the evidence?
Could I be making a mistake in the way I am thinking?
Am I thinking straight?
Am I pressurizing myself?
Am I using the language of the extremist?
What is the worst thing that could happen?

Step 5: Come up with an alternative, balanced thought

'I can't do this.' Having difficulties with sex is common for people
  with diabetes.
'It's not working as it should.' I won't always have this struggle.
'This is embarrassing.' I'm following a plan and learning how to enjoy
  sex again.
'I'll never be normal.' I'm getting control over the problem, by
  implementing this plan. I'm going to ask Francesca to compliment
  me/my appearance when we are in bed together.
'Francesca will think I don't love her or I don't find her attractive any
  more.' I'm going to focus on *all* the aspects of the sexual experience:
  the closeness and intimacy with Francesca, how good it feels to be
  touched, how nice it is to be kissed and stroked.
Every time I am aware of the anxiety I have in relation to sex, and
  think of these alternative thoughts, I am getting better.

Kindness statement

Use your thinking in step 5 to formulate a 'kindness statement' and
keep it somewhere convenient (in your diary or bag or by your bed)
and read it at least three times a day to help keep these new thoughts
close to hand.

References

Anderson, Robert and Funnell, Martha (2005). Patient empowerment: reflections on the challenge of fostering the adoption of a new paradigm. *Patient Education and Counselling*, 57, 153–7.
Chapman, Gary (1992). *The Five Love Languages*. Moody, Chicago, IL.
Diabetes UK (2008). Minding the gap: the provision of psychological support and care for people with diabetes in the UK. www.diabetes.org.uk/Documents /Reports/Minding_the_Gap_psychological_report.pdf. Accessed April 2008.
Ford, Vicki (2005). *Overcoming Sexual Problems*. Constable and Robinson, London.
Polonsky, William (1999). *Diabetes Burnout*. American Diabetes Association. Alexandria, VA.

Further Reading

Linda Blair (2008). *Straight Talking*. Piatkus, London.
Gillian Butler and Tony Hope (1995). *Manage Your Mind*. Oxford University Press, Oxford.
Gary Chapman (1992). *The Five Love Languages*. Moody, Chicago, IL.
Vicki Ford (2005). *Overcoming Sexual Problems*. Constable and Robinson, London.
William Polonsky (1999). *Diabetes Burnout*. American Diabetes Association, Alexandria, VA.

8

Implementing Change

This book is all about making changes to your life with diabetes. It is one thing knowing what changes you would like to make; it is quite another to actually be able to implement them. This chapter and the next help you to put your plans into action. Change is often related to the concept of motivation, so this chapter begins by discussing the often paradoxical nature of the concept of motivation and then describes a seven-step plan for implementing change.

The Paradox of Motivation

I have lost count of the times people with diabetes have said to me, 'I would love to change my behaviour around diabetes, but I just have no motivation.' They know *what* they should be doing to care for their health, but they cannot seem to summon up the *how*. So when I tell them, 'You are one of the most motivated people I have ever seen', they tend to stare at me in utter disbelief! But then I explain. They are motivated to do all sorts of things in life:

Watch the latest film at the cinema.
Devote some time to engaging in an enjoyable pastime or hobby.
Pet their cat or dog.
Eat a delicious meal in the company of loved ones.
Go on holiday.

I am confident there is not a single person reading this who finds that the concept of 'motivation' enters their mind when they are thinking of

Diabetes and Wellbeing: Managing the Psychological and Emotional Challenges of Diabetes Types 1 and 2, First Edition. Dr Jen Nash.
© 2013 John Wiley & Sons, Ltd. Published 2013 by John Wiley & Sons, Ltd.

doing these fun activities. In fact, the average person would be ready, willing and eager to get started and feel the enjoyment that these events bring.

The crucial difference with these things is that they are a short-term route to good feelings and instant pleasure. The problem with health-promoting activities such as exercising, eating healthily or testing your blood glucose is that they often do not result in pleasure in the short term: instead working up a sweat is uncomfortable, the salads are more boring than the chips, and testing your blood glucose is more pain than it is worth.

No one feels motivated to do something if the costs seem to outweigh the benefits. Go to the gym in the evening or spend a cosy night in front of the television? I am sure you can see what I mean.

Here are my top tips for staying motivated with any aspect of your diabetes health care:

Link an activity that feels like a struggle with one that naturally feels effortless

You could:

test your blood glucose and then phone or email a friend you love to chat to straight after;

plan your exercise so it's immediately followed by watching your favourite TV programme;

make the doctor's appointment you have been putting off for months just before you sit down with your morning tea or coffee, and make a rule that you can't have one until you've done it;

stick to your healthy eating plan for three days and reward yourself with a visit to your favourite museum, gallery, park or shop.

Imagine, and keep imagining, how great you will feel once you've accomplished your goal

The goal may be losing a certain amount of weight, getting to the HbA1c level you are aiming for, or engaging in a regular routine of exercising more. Having a photo, picture or object that symbolizes or is a reminder of your goal can be effective when you feel you are losing motivation, perhaps because your goal is taking too long or the results seem too slow.

Kindness statement

Keep your inner voice kind and supportive. It is so easy to find yourself talking to yourself in a negative way, and, even worse, listening to it. Form a kindness statement that you find motivating and remind yourself of it often. Examples are: 'If this was easy, everyone would be doing it!', 'Only I can change my life. No one can do it for me', 'Change is challenging but each day I'm moving closer to my desired goal'.

Remind yourself of things you have achieved in the past

Think how you can transfer this experience to your current goal.

Keep a success journal and track all of your successes, no matter how small or in what area of life. Examples could be: learning to drive, making a new friend or nurturing an existing relationship, learning how to use a computer, raising your child, having a successful work meeting, learning a new recipe, mastering a new skill, planning a holiday or family day out . . . you get the idea!

You might like to think back over times you have changed in the past and fill in the following worksheet.

Example worksheet: learning from change

Change I want to make
Lose one stone in weight by avoiding snacking between meals

What are your main reasons for making this change?
Feel fitter, look better, be healthier

Thinking over times you have made a health change in the past, how did you do it?
Cut out sugar in my tea – ensured I didn't have any in the house, kept reminders by the kettle

What helped you to stay on track?
Telling others of my plans, talking to other non-sugar takers and seeing what their experiences were like

---

What things got in your way?

Going to a friend's house – had to remember to tell her I no longer took sugar

Which strategies were the most successful?

Using a sugar substitute when I really fancied some sweetness

How will you respond to the urge to go back to an old behaviour?

Remind myself of how good it will feel to succeed this time, distract myself with an activity

How do you expect to feel when you have succeeded?

Fantastic!

What might you miss about your old behaviour?

Having a cake with tea when I meet a friend. I could plan to buy myself a non-food treat instead, e.g. a magazine or a new product I have not tried before

Have you told people about your plans? If not, why not?

No, will tell my partner and ask her for support

Can you think up some responses you can give if tempted to stray from your plans?

'I'm really enjoying feeling more in control of my health'

Are there any friendships that may be affected when you make this change?

Mum might be a bit miffed if I don't eat snacks she has made when I visit her. I could always ask her to wrap it up and tell her I will eat it later, or share it with my partner.

Worksheet: Learning From Change

Change I want to make

What is your main reason for making this change?

Thinking over times you've made a health change in the past, how did you do it?

What helped you to stay on track?

What things got in your way?

Which strategies were the most successful?

How will you respond to the urge to go back to an old behaviour?

How do you expect to feel when you have succeeded?

What might you miss about your old behaviour?

Have you told people about your plans? If not, why not?

Can you think up some responses you can give if tempted to stray from your plans?

Are there any friendships that may be affected when you make this change?

Seven-Step Plan for Implementing Change

Step 1: Set a goal

Setting goals is a crucial part of making any change in your life. The self-help author Zig Ziglar was once quoted as saying that people tend not to wander around and then suddenly find themselves at the top of Mount Everest. Earl Nightingale, author of a short text, *The Strangest Secret*, labelled one of the best motivational books of all time, talks of the importance of goal setting, likening our lives to a ship that leaves a harbour: with a map, destination and crew, the ship will reach its destination 99 per cent of the time. Without the map, destination and crew, if it does manage to leave the harbour it will either sink or end up derelict on a deserted beach. It cannot go anywhere without a destination or guidance. It is the same with a human being.

Even if you are someone who does not think of your life in terms of goals set and achieved, I can assure you that you do make use of them, and probably very often; it is just you are not explicitly aware of them. You bought or picked up this book with the goal of learning more about the psychology of diabetes. You went to bed last night with the goal of falling asleep. You ate a meal today with the goal of satisfying your hunger. You applied for a job with the goal of getting it. You cuddled your child with the goal of soothing their upset. Goals make up every aspect of your life and are an important aspect of making any significant change in life. Goals need to be specific and concrete. In the same way as travelling to a destination requires a full address, having a specific plan of what your life will look like once your goal is achieved is crucial. Begin with the end in mind.

To help you with your goal setting, you can use the SMART process. SMART is an acronym for the different aspects that are involved in setting a goal that works.

Specific: The goal is well defined
Measurable: The goal can be tangibly measured by an outside observer
Attainable: The goal is attainable and achievable
Realistic: The goal is within the availability of resources, money and time
Time-bound: There is a time limit to the goal (enough time to achieve it, but not too much time, as this can be counter-productive)

For example:

'To lose weight' is a goal
'To weigh 10 stone by 31 December this year' is a SMART goal, as it includes
the five elements listed above.

Let's look at each of these factors in more detail.

Specific

Rather than simply stating a general goal such as 'I want to lose weight' or 'I want to exercise more', it is important to be very specific. If you just say that your goal is 'to lose weight', then you have achieved this goal whether you have lost one kilogram or twenty. Being specific is crucial, because it allows you to measure your progress to success and is a clear indicator of whether or not you have met the goal you set yourself.

Measurable

It is important that you can objectively observe whether you have reached the goal or not. In the case of a weight-loss goal, the weighing scales or your body measurements will show whether or not you've achieved the goal. By weighing yourself and measuring the circumference of your waist, hips, thighs, arms and so on you can gather objective, observable evidence based on fact, not just your feelings, which can often be inaccurate. Likewise, if you want to test your blood glucose more frequently and your goal is to test twice per day, someone else can objectively witness the achievement or non-achievement of this goal.

Attainable

The goal needs to be achievable to ensure you do not set a goal that is impossible to meet, which would reinforce a sense of failure. For example, if your goal is to lose a specified amount of weight, you may need to get some help from your healthcare team to decide whether it is indeed an achievable goal given your current circumstances. If you have a lot of weight to lose, you may need to break down this large overall goal into smaller goals to help you stay on track, taking it one stone or ten kilograms at a time, for example. You also need to consider your personal circumstances. If your goal is to test your blood glucose three times a day but you currently never test and have a family of young children to care for, a more achievable goal to begin with may be to test once a day. Remember that goals can always be reviewed and updated at a later stage.

Realistic

Although thinking big and aiming high can be motivating, it is also important to be realistic with goal setting. Feeling good about taking 'baby steps' towards your goal is important. Although small steps can sometimes seem insignificant when you have many changes to make, they are easier to accomplish and will not move you too far out of your current comfort zone, which is important if you are to avoid overwhelm. However, when viewed over the course of a week, a month, three months, six months, or a year, all of those baby steps in the right direction will have had a significant cumulative effect. So, for example, if one of your actions is to cut out the biscuit you always eat with your mid-morning cup of tea, it might seem like a very small change but over the course of the year it is likely to show a really dramatic difference on the weighing scales.

Time-bound

It is crucial to have a time by which you will achieve the goal, to help you to maintain momentum. You might like to set the goal for a particular event such as a holiday or your birthday: for example, 'By my birthday I will be feeling fantastic at 10 stone 5 pounds.' However, avoid this if it means rushing for the deadline. It is also important to take it slowly and be patient. Change is challenging and many people get frustrated and want to see results straight away – overnight if possible! However, the reality is that it is likely that the problem you are working on has become a problem over a long period of time. Just as the problem has arisen in a small and steady way, it will be solved in a slow and steady way. A good example of this may be weight gain, in which eating a relatively small number of additional calories each day can add up to a large difference on the scales over time. It is important to emphasize that, although you may need to be patient at first, as with everything in life if you take consistent action on your goals you will get the desired result in the end. In just the same way as you learned how to drive a car or use the internet, you got better with time and practice. The advantage of this is that, because it is a lifestyle change rather than a quick fix, you will be able to improve your health in a much more sustainable and long-lasting way.

Take a moment now to write out the next goal you plan to action, ensuring it is as SMART as possible.

SMART goal
Specific
Measurable
Attainable
Realistic
Time-bound
My SMART goal is

Step 2: Make a plan

Wiseman (2009) has a simple process for making plans that work. Break your overall SMART goal into a maximum of five smaller steps. Each step should also be a goal that is SMART. Think about how you will achieve each sub-goal, and the reward you will give yourself when you complete it.

Step 1
My first sub-goal is:
I believe I can achieve this goal because:
To achieve this sub-goal I will:
This will be achieved by the following date:
My reward for achieving this will be:

Step 2

My second sub-goal is:

I believe I can achieve this goal because:

To achieve this sub-goal I will:

This will be achieved by the following date:

My reward for achieving this will be:

Step 3

My third sub-goal is:

I believe I can achieve this goal because:

To achieve this sub-goal I will:

This will be achieved by the following date:

My reward for achieving this will be:

Step 4

My fourth sub-goal is:

I believe I can achieve this goal because:

To achieve this sub-goal I will:

This will be achieved by the following date:

My reward for achieving this will be:

Step 5

My fifth sub-goal is:

I believe I can achieve this goal because:

To achieve this sub-goal I will:

This will be achieved by the following date:

My reward for achieving this will be:

Step 3: Go public

People who successfully reach their goals are far more likely to have told their friends, family and/or colleagues about their intentions. Although keeping your goals private can help you avoid looking foolish if you do not manage to reach them, it also makes it very tempting to avoid making the life changes you need and consequently return to your usual routines and habits. This is true for much of human behaviour. In one classic psychology experiment, students were shown some lines that had been drawn on a board and were asked to estimate their length. Those that made a public commitment to their judgement by writing their decision down and sharing it with the group were much more likely to stand by their opinion when they were told it might be wrong than those who had kept their estimate private (Deutsch & Gerard, 1955).

Another important benefit of going public is that friends and family can actually help you to achieve your goals by offering encouragement and support when you are struggling. This is one reason why weight loss groups and twelve-step addiction recovery programmes can be helpful. Knowing you are not alone and having people to pick you up when you need it is important.

A word of caution, though. Be thoughtful about who you tell. You do not have to go public with everyone you know, particularly if there are some people in your life who may have a vested interest in you *not* changing. Remember that when you make a change, it can shine a light on others, who may examine their own lives and find that they fall short. If you can change, then they have proof that they could too, which can sometimes be an uncomfortable realization.

Make a list of the people you know who can support you:

_____

_____

_____

_____

_____

_____

Step 4: Link pleasure to goal achievement

Individuals who maintain their consistency towards goal achievement tend to remind themselves frequently of the benefits of reaching their desired outcome. Many self-help books advise you to imagine your desired future self, but this strategy can fail if the individual isn't able to also change their internal identity to this future 'perfect' (unrealistic) version of themselves. A better strategy is to make a reality-based checklist of how your experience of daily life will improve once you have achieved your goal. List these in terms of the advantages of your anticipated future, rather than avoiding the undesirable features of your existing situation. For example, 'I'll be able to play football with the children' rather than, 'The children won't tire me out so quickly.' A subtle but important shift in emphasis.

Benefit 1: _____

Benefit 2: _____

Benefit 3: _____

Step 5: Reward yourself

Have you ever made a New Year's Resolution that was a distant memory by February? I thought so! Many people make commitments to make a change in their life, but not everyone actually manages to reach their goal. What is the difference between those who achieve success and those who do not? Goal achievement is a huge area of study in psychology and there are an enormous array of factors that contribute to successfully achieving plans and goals. However, one key component that is consistently demonstrated to be important is the use of rewards.

If you think back over the last couple of days, it's likely that virtually every task or activity that you successfully completed had some benefit or payoff – in other words, a reward. You cooked a meal in order to enjoy the reward of eating it. You went to work to gain the reward of getting paid (and hopefully obtaining some level of enjoyment!). You gave directions to a lost stranger to receive the reward of feeling that you had done a good deed. You did the gardening to achieve the reward of your environment looking better. You may have left your waiter or waitress at the restaurant a tip, not just because of the service they provided but also because you desired the reward of feeling that you were socially acceptable. Take a moment now to think back over the things you've done in the last week and list some of the rewards, both obvious and implied, that you received for engaging in them.

Recent ways I have been rewarded:

_____

_____

_____

_____

_____

_____

_____

_____

_____

The link between actions and rewards begins very early on in life. Infants are rewarded for their tears by their mother's milk or the feeling of relief from a wet nappy. Children enjoy the praise and attention they receive when they take their first steps, the new toy they receive when their school report card is good and the hug their mother gives them when they behave well at an important event. Adolescents are very motivated to wear the 'right' clothes in order to fit in with their peers. Some are motivated to study hard at school and college for the reward of good grades and a promising career, while others are motivated to avoid academic work in order to gain relief from having to try and perhaps still fail, or to fit in with their peer group. Do you see how the concept of rewards is a very personal and complex one?

In the same way, you can be thoughtful about the kinds of rewards and payoffs that you find motivating, which are likely to be unique to you and completely different from others around you. You can use this knowledge and insight to help you stay on track with your diabetes-related goals.

Spend some time now reflecting on the kinds of activities you currently find rewarding and pleasurable and list them below. Here are some ideas to help you:

Listening to music
Shopping
Smoking
Spending time with friends

Watching TV
Going to the cinema
Exercising
Drinking alcohol
Surfing the Internet
Reading
Playing sports
Taking drugs
Eating chocolate
Watching a film
Dancing
Taking a walk
Going to a party

_____

_____

_____

_____

_____

_____

_____

_____

_____

Be honest and write everything down. Do not censor yourself; no one has to see the list except you! Whilst all of these activities are rewarding in their own way, some are more helpful than others. If you wrote down that your favourite rewards involve chocolate and alcohol, and you engage in these regularly, your health will be at risk. Whilst these rewards can be used in moderation, it will help you to develop a larger repertoire of alternatives to engage in. Here are some ideas to start you off.

Pet a cat or dog
Have a lie-down or a nap
Do a jigsaw puzzle
Plan a holiday
Read a book
Write a letter

Window-shop
Rearrange the furniture
Go for a walk
Feed the birds
Plant something
Buy flowers for yourself or someone else
Clean your car or your bike
Go online and research something new
Mend something
Phone a friend
Go to a museum
Introduce yourself to a neighbour
Organize your wardrobe
Visit the library
Watch the sunset
Send a card
Start a new evening class
Buy a magazine
Clean something
Sort out a drawer
Play solitaire
Arrange a date
Enter a competition
Go for a picnic
Plan an outing on your next free day
Stick some photos in an album
Learn a new language
Volunteer for a charity
Do some gardening
Visit a new town
See a movie
Play an instrument
Praise yourself, e.g. 'Well done!' and 'I'm doing great!'
Give a massage
Send an e-mail
Check your bank statement
Go swimming
Polish some silver or brass
Research a political party
Make a list of everything you want to do next year

Draw or paint a picture
Clear out a cupboard
Do some sport
Water your plants

Use the space below to add your own ideas.

_____

_____

_____

_____

_____

_____

_____

_____

_____

Rewards can be symbolic, they don't have to involve spending money. Often it is the timing that's important. For example, you could plan to watch your favourite TV programme after you have been out for the brisk walk you are not looking forward to. Arrange to chat on the phone to a friend after you have tested your blood glucose rather than before, or perhaps plan to have that mid-morning cup of tea after you have chatted to your diabetes nurse or had a hospital appointment. Alternatively, you could design a system in which you exchange tokens for rewards: award yourself one token for each challenging activity you engage in, and after 5 or 10 tokens (you decide), 'exchange' these tokens for a CD, a new item of clothing, some fresh flowers . . . again, you decide!

Change can be challenging, and by its very nature it moves you beyond your comfort zone. Making changes can feel difficult and you may encounter some resistance when you are trying to achieve your goal; this is natural. So, to keep yourself motivated, it is important to reward yourself for achieving certain milestones. Rewards are a good way to give yourself the extra push you might need to do something that feels difficult.

These are just ideas to start you off. You know yourself best and the kinds of activities that will act as motivating rewards to help you achieve your goals when things are feeling challenging. Why not prepare a list of your top ten rewards below, and enjoy not only engaging in them, but also moving ever closer to the health and wellbeing you want with each one?

My top ten rewards

1	
2	
3	
4	
5	
6	
7	
8	
9	
10	

Step 6: Update your identity

Life is full of activity, demands and commitments that can become distractions from your goals if you let them. In order to sustain progress towards your aims, it is crucial to keep your desired goal uppermost in your mind.

In order to do this, it can help to surround yourself with some tangible reminders of your goal. Below are some ideas you could try.

An image that represents your dream goal

A photo of your ideal figure from a magazine
The medal you will achieve when you complete your fitness goal
A photo of yourself at your dream weight
A 'Dream Book': a journal or scrapbook with blank pages in which you
    can depict a series of goals and dreams using pictures from magazines
    or whatever suits you. Each page could have a different dream category:
    weight, eating habits, blood glucose levels, relationships with healthcare
    team, relationships with loved ones, etc.

Using your imagination   Imagining yourself living the life of your dreams can be extremely motivating. Spend time each day using your imagination in this way, perhaps when you are doing something else that you find relaxing, such as taking a shower or a bath, or before you go to bed. Focus particularly on the advantages that this future way of living will bring in comparison to your current life: how will you feel, what exciting things will fill your days, what current stresses will you be free of?

Updating my identity

_____

_____

_____

_____

_____

_____

_____

_____

Step 7: Get started now

The final important point about goal setting is to focus on immediate action. Therefore, as soon as you have finished reading this page, I want you to write down something that you can do today: some very small task that will get you moving towards progress and a different future for yourself. It could be something like spending five minutes before the end of the day reviewing your goals, making a healthy choice at dinner, making sure your blood glucose testing kit is in order, whatever is relevant to your goal. It does not need to be something that requires a complete overhaul of your usual routine, but rather some small action that you can take with relative ease to symbolize that you are starting afresh with a new sense of purpose towards your goals. Using Table 8.1 as a model, write it in Table 8.2.

It's easy to see that by just completing small actions daily, weekly and monthly you will be moving ever closer to your goal. The momentum of achieving progress on your goals in this way can be very motivating.

Table 8.1 Example first steps towards change

Goal	Small steps to move me towards this goal	Deadline to achieve it by
Begin to test my blood glucose	Doing research on the Internet into the pros and cons of different testing equipment	Tuesday
	Talking to someone with diabetes (perhaps virtually, on a diabetes internet forum) about their experiences	
Gain confidence in talking to my doctor about diabetes	Borrow a book from the public library about communication skills	Go to the library on Saturday
	Write down the main points of what I want to say and role-play the conversation with a family member/friend	The end of the month [state specific date]

Table 8.2 First steps towards change

Goal	Small steps to move me towards this goal	Deadline to achieve it by

References

Deutsch, M. and Gerard, H. (1955). A study of normative and informational social influences upon individual judgment. *Journal of Abnormal and Social Psychology*, 51, 629–36.

Wiseman, R. (2009). *59 Seconds: Think a Little, Change a Lot*. Macmillan, London.

Further Reading

J. Canfield and J. Switzer (2005). *The Success Principles: How to Get From Where You Are to Where You Want to Be*. Element, London.

F. Harrold (2001). *Be Your Own Life Coach: How to Take Control of Your Life and Achieve Your Wildest Dreams*. Coronet Books, London.

Earl Nightingale (2006). *The Strangest Secret*. BN Publishing, Thousand Oaks, CA.

J. Olson (2005). *The Slight Edge: Secret to a Successful Life*. Success Books, Lake Dallas, TX.

A. Robbins (1997). *Awaken the Giant Within*. Simon and Schuster, London.

Richard Wiseman (2009). *59 Seconds: Think a Little, Change a Lot*. Macmillan, London.

9

Managing Setbacks, Staying Solution-Focused and Embracing Mindfulness

Setbacks are inevitable. I applaud you for reading this book and making plans to change your relationship with diabetes, and I give you full permission to make mistakes and get a bit off track every now and then. These experiences are paradoxically a crucial component of long-term success. Confused? All will be explained in this chapter, and advice will be given about how to stay solution-focused to maintain progress.

We live in a success-addicted society where anything other than one hundred per cent perfection can be shunned, leading to a polarized experience of 'good', or 'bad'. However, extensive research into the principles of successful people and outcomes demonstrates that success is a steady process of moving forward despite (or even because of) the need to face, tackle and overcome challenges that might get in the way of progress. A helpful analogy is that of the pilot who spends a large percentage of the flying time off the flight path, but with a process of constant course correction can successfully reach the target destination. In the same way, you need to be a flexible pilot of your diabetes, actively embracing and encouraging setbacks throughout the change process. It is only by tackling setbacks and correcting your course that you can be confident that the change you have made is a lasting one.

Diabetes and Wellbeing: Managing the Psychological and Emotional Challenges of Diabetes Types 1 and 2, First Edition. Dr Jen Nash.
© 2013 John Wiley & Sons, Ltd. Published 2013 by John Wiley & Sons, Ltd.

Learn the Difference Between a Lapse and a Relapse

As discussed in previous chapters, the first step is to know the difference between a lapse and a relapse. A lapse occurs when you go off track temporarily, for example by eating the dessert you were not planning on having, missing an exercise session or avoiding testing your blood glucose for a day. Lapses are not failures: they are an inevitable and often helpful part of changing behaviour. We need to have times when we go off track in order to help us problem-solve for next time.

A relapse happens when you allow a string of lapses to overwhelm you without taking corrective action. 'All-or-nothing thinking', the belief that you are being either completely 'good' or completely 'bad', can really get in your way when it comes to reaching your goals. No matter how well you think you are doing, there will always be some obstacles in your way. Yes, you will make mistakes and get off track – that is life – but the secret is to learn from them and carry on despite them.

In considering recovery from addictions, people often talk about relapsing. One definition of a relapse is 'a deterioration in health after a temporary improvement'. A lapse, on the other hand is, 'a temporary failure of concentration, memory, or judgement'. The key word here is 'temporary'. Many people get off track with change: this is what we call a lapse. It is only when a number of lapses are strung together in a row that we would call it a relapse. What is important is to identify a lapse and stop it in its tracks by getting back on course to goal fulfilment.

Many people fall into the cognitive distortion of all-or-nothing thinking in relation to lapses, and attribute it to a personal failure rather than just a one-off event or an environmental challenge. It is demanding for even the most motivated person to stay on track with the weight loss goal when at a birthday party full of sweet and fattening food.

The important step is to review and take stock of each lapse as it occurs and problem-solve in the following way.

Example: Learning from a lapse

What happened?

I overate at my friend's birthday party.

Why did it happen?

I was hungry and there were only unhealthy foods available.

If I was in the same situation again what would I do differently?

Eat a snack before I leave the house.
Bring some healthy foods along with me.
Keep away from the room where the food is served.
Forgive myself, it's a party!

Learning from a lapse

What happened?

Why did it happen?

If I was in the same situation again what would I do differently?

In this way, lapses become good opportunities for learning about making and sustaining changes in the 'real world'. This is precisely the reason why some people struggling with addictions lapse when they leave the safety of the detox setting and return to their usual environment. It is not simply a matter of losing motivation or willpower, but of facing and dealing with the everyday challenges that will inevitably arise.

It is likely that some people reading this will have got to the point of a relapse. In which case, well done for continuing with this chapter! That in itself is a success. Let's take stock. How far did you get with your progress before you slipped? Take a minute now to list below any changes you made before the relapse, no matter how small or insignificant you might think they were.

_____

_____

_____

_____

_____

_____

_____

_____

Recognize and value the progress you made, and remember that if you have done it once you can do it again!

Staying Solution-Focused

A useful way of tackling problems and obstacles to progress when they inevitably arise is to use a solution-focused approach. Rather than focusing on and analysing the problem in order to find a resolution, solution-focused approaches emphasize what is going well, with attention placed on repeating and building on these successes, no matter how small they may seem (de Shazer, 1988). Whatever the challenge there are always times when the problem is a little less difficult than usual or the difficulty is not affecting you quite so much. This approach encourages you to describe what the different circumstances were in that case, or what you did differently. By examining the situation from this perspective, you can repeat what has worked in the past, and gain confidence in your ability to make improvements for the future.

Looking for exceptions

Bring to mind a goal you have in relation to your diabetes, perhaps one you are struggling with. Think back over the last week or two and recall if there was a day, or even a moment in the day, when you were feeling a bit more in control in this area. What was different about that day? When in the day did you feel this sense of control? Where were you? Who were you with? You will see that aspects of your preferred future are already occurring; it is just difficult to keep these in mind when you think globally about your problem.

Using the miracle question

Suppose you were to put this book down and do whatever you planned to do for the rest of the day. Then, sometime in the evening, you get tired and go to sleep. In the middle of the night, when you are fast asleep, a miracle happens and all the problems that brought you to this book today are solved 'just like that'. When you wake up the next morning, how are you going to start discovering that the miracle happened?' (de Shazer, 1988)

What will you notice?
What else?
What will be different?
What else?
How will others be reacting to you?
How else?

For many people their first response is, 'I don't know!' This is because we hardly ever look at life in this way, so it can feel rather strange at first. However, if you can overcome your resistance and give yourself time to fully absorb the question, you can begin to see what your preferred future looks like.

Scaling

Once the miracle day has been thoroughly explored, give today a rating in relation to it on a scale of 0–10, where 0 is the worst things have ever been and 10 is the miracle day.

Whatever number you give yourself for today, ask yourself the following questions (de Shazer, 1988):

What will be the first thing that will let you know you are one point higher?
What is stopping you from slipping one point lower down the scale?

On a day when you are one point higher on the scale, what would tell you that it was a 'one point higher' day?

Where on the scale would be good enough? What would a day at that point on the scale look like?

What have you done to prevent things being worse?

How did you do that?

In what ways was that helpful?

What do you think you would want to continue doing to get that to happen more often?

If you give your day a 0, or even a negative number, why have you not yet given up and are still prepared to read this book? What has prevented things from getting even worse?

This approach helps you to identify times in your current life that are closer to this ideal future, and to examine what is different on these occasions. It brings these small successes to your awareness and helps you to repeat these successful things that you do when the problem is not there or less severe, so that you can move towards the ideal future you have identified.

Case study: Mahesh

Mahesh is struggling with emotional eating. When she is upset she has a tendency to snack on biscuits and sweets to cheer herself up.

Q: 'If you woke up tomorrow, and a miracle happened so that you no longer reached for the biscuit tin when you felt emotional, what would be different? What would the first signs be that the miracle had occurred?'

A: 'I wouldn't be reaching for the biscuits when I have an argument with my partner.'

Q: 'What will you be doing instead when you have an argument with your partner?'

A: 'I will be talking to him calmly about the way that I feel. I can see myself going for a walk, listening to music or writing my feelings in a letter.'

Q: 'How can you use this knowledge to help you?'

A: 'I could ask my partner if we could try talking calmly rather than arguing. I could put a post-it note on the biscuit tin, with bullet points to remind me of these ideas. I could create a playlist of my favourite music to play when we have had a disagreement.'

Acceptance and Mindfulness

One of the biggest challenges of diabetes is to accept the inevitability that it will be a part of your life for the foreseeable future. Much of the discussion and many of the CBT strategies in this book encourage change and a move towards doing things differently. Although much of our inner thought and emotional life can be changed for the better, an element of acknowledgement is needed that diabetes cannot be altered and does need to be accepted. An approach called *mindfulness* can assist with the process of greater acceptance. This part of the chapter will describe mindfulness and how you can implement it into your life.

What is mindfulness?

Mindfulness is simply a commitment to live in the moment. Put in a broader way, mindfulness is the awareness that arises from paying attention on purpose, in the present moment, non-judgementally, to things as they are (Williams, Teasdale, Segal and Kabat-Zinn, 2007). For many of us, our attention and thoughts are focused on the past, on memories or regrets; or on the future, on anxiety or uncertainty about what is to come. However, in reality, the only moment we truly have is the one occurring right now. Mindfulness encourages you to focus on the here and now, and let go of thoughts of the past and future. It is not about paying more attention so much as paying attention in a different and wiser way, with the whole mind and senses at work. Developing a capacity to live in the moment can be enormously freeing. If, while working through this chapter, you have found it difficult to let go of regret about something you have not done as well as you could (such as the food choices you've made), or if you find yourself continually dwelling on the possibility of developing complications, for example, then you will probably find mindfulness will help.

Mindfulness and CBT

Like CBT, mindfulness involves paying attention to your internal experiences, such as your thoughts and emotions. However, in contrast to CBT, mindfulness does not encourage you to change these thoughts and emotions. Rather, it urges you to simply notice the thoughts you are having, rather than actively engage in them. Thoughts stream rapidly through our minds and mindfulness encourages us to sit back and 'observe' our thoughts, rather than becoming involved in them. While the techniques in this book have encouraged you to engage with your inner thinking life by challenging those thoughts that don't serve you, mindfulness encourages you to view thoughts as inner experiences that do not actually need to be engaged in at all.

For example, imagine a book beside you right now, perhaps called *Mindfulness for Diabetes*, with a picture of a sturdy oak tree on the front of it. You will (hopefully!) be able to distinguish this imagined book from the very real book you are now holding in your hands as you are reading it. This is easy because one is physically tangible – you are touching it – and one is the product of your imagination. However, when your mind offers you thoughts about things that are not physically tangible to begin with, like your worth as a person with diabetes, it can be harder to distinguish how 'real' they are. Actually, a thought such as 'I am rubbish at taking care of my diabetes' is no different to the thought of the imaginary book. It is not a fact, simply a thought. The difference is that we tend to quickly shift our attention from thoughts of imaginary books, as there is likely to be little if any emotion or feeling attached to them. A self-critical thought usually does cause a shift in mood. Mindfulness can help you see how the experience just fades when you do not engage with the feeling element of unhelpful thoughts.

Mindfulness and diabetes

Research studies have shown that regular practice of mindfulness helps those with type 1 and type 2 better manage their difficult emotions about diabetes and also has a positive impact on their blood glucose control. Furthermore, it is a practice that is pretty straightforward to learn and implement. Rosenzweig, Reibel, Greeson, Edman et al. (2007) found that HbA1c, depression and anxiety were decreased among patients with type 2 diabetes who participated in a standard Mindfulness-Based Stress Reduction programme.

Box 9.1 An exercise in mindful eating

A wonderfully simple way of having a taste (literally!) of mindfulness is to eat a raisin. You are probably thinking, 'Eat one raisin? I couldn't eat just one!' Try this exercise (Williams, Teasdale, Segal and Kabat-Zinn, 2007) and you might be surprised.

Holding

Take a raisin and hold it between your finger and thumb or in the palm of your hand. Imagine you are a visitor to this planet and have never seen a raisin before, or anything like it. Focus on this new object with fresh eyes.

Seeing

Gaze at the raisin for a while with your full attention, examining every single aspect and feature of its ridges, folds and hollows.

Touching

Concentrate on its texture and move it between your fingers. How does it feel against your skin?

Smelling

Bring the raisin to your nose and notice any smell or fragrance you can ascertain. Attend to your mouth and stomach and anything occurring there.

Placing

Move your hand up to your mouth and place it on your tongue. Explore how it feels as it rests there.

Tasting

Take a bite into the raisin and concentrate on how the taste is experienced in your mouth. Notice how this changes moment by moment. Bite again and see if the taste changes.

Swallowing

When you are ready, prepare to swallow the raisin. Notice there is an intention to swallow before you actually do.

Following

See if you can feel the raisin move down your throat and into your stomach. Notice how your body is feeling now you have eaten in this mindful way.

Record your observations here.

_____

_____

_____

_____

_____

_____

_____

_____

_____

A mindfulness exercise

Once you have had an experience of mindful eating (Box 9.1), you can move on to try a 10-minute mindfulness exercise (Williams, Teasdale, Segal and Kabat-Zinn, 2007).

1. Settle into a comfortable sitting position in a chair, with your feet flat on the floor and legs uncrossed. If you would like to close your eyes then do so, but it is not necessary. If you are more comfortable with your eyes open then cast an unfocused gaze on the floor a few feet in front of you.
2. Begin by noticing the points of your body that are in contact with the chair. Observe the feeling of touch and pressure, in your hands and arms, your back, buttocks, thighs and anywhere else you are in contact with the chair. Take a minute or two to do this.
3. Now notice your breathing: the movement in your stomach and chest region, and the sensation in your nostrils. Once you have spent a few

moments focusing on each of these in turn, pick the area that feels most vivid to you, to concentrate on. Notice the changing physical sensation on the in-breath and out-breath and the slight pauses that occur between them. There is no need to attempt to change or control your natural breathing in any way. There is no striving for a particular way of being to be achieved.

4. At some point in this process your mind will do what it does best – wander! Perhaps you will notice you are no longer thinking about the sensation of breathing, but wondering what to have for dinner, day-dreaming about the weekend, worrying about your work presentation in the morning or noticing you have an itch in your elbow. This is not a sign you are failing at the task, or you have made a mistake. To the contrary, it is to be celebrated: as soon as you have noticed your attention has gone elsewhere you are back on the path to refocusing on the sensation of breathing. Be kind to yourself and observe, 'Oh look, my mind has wandered . . . let me just bring it back to my breathing.'

5. Your mind will continue to pull your thoughts onto these distractions. That is OK. It can be a bit of a to-and-fro experience; however, let it be just this: a to and fro of gently noticing and pulling back your attention to your breath, rather than a struggling 'push-pull' type of back-and-forth experience. Be a kind mother or father (rather than a strict and controlling one) to your thoughts, gently steering them where you want them to be. Remind yourself that the intention is simply to be aware of your moment-to-moment experience, whatever the experience is, as best you can. Continue this practice for 10 minutes, or longer if you would like to

Once you have completed this 10-minute exercise, what do you notice? You might notice your mind calming and your thoughts becoming a little less stressful. In addition, focusing on something external to yourself, rather than the internal voice of your thoughts, can be helpful. This can be as simple as the sensation of your hands against the paper you are holding, or your breathing, or how it feels to sit in the chair you are in; where is the tension held in your body? This can feel strange and difficult at first, but with practice it can lead to a more peaceful experience of daily life.

How to use mindfulness with difficult feelings about diabetes

Use the exercise above for a few minutes to get in a place of readiness for this exercise.

When you are ready and are feeling a bit more relaxed, bring to mind a difficult emotion that you're aware of in relation to your diabetes. Start with the one that feels the easiest. It may be frustration, fear, anxiety, guilt, shame, resentment, depression or something else. Start with whatever emotion is right for you: something unresolved or a bit unpleasant.

Once you have begun to focus on this feeling, become aware of your body and any physical feelings that are occurring for you when you bring this feeling into awareness. Deliberately shift your focus to the part of your body where the physical sensation is the strongest.

Welcome it, by imagining you are breathing into it. Accept it by saying to yourself, 'It's OK. This feeling is here right now. Let me open to it.'

Stay loose and soft and let go of any tension or rigidity you might be aware of. You are not judging the feeling, or saying that everything is fine, or trying to fix it; you are simply allowing it to be.

When you notice that the bodily symptoms are no longer pulling you in the same way or to the same intensity, simply shift your attention back to your breathing in the way you were doing at the start of the exercise.

How to use mindfulness in everyday life

The real value of practising mindfulness comes when you can bring the skills developed in these two exercises into your daily life.

Bring moment-to-moment awareness to routine activities such as showering, brushing your teeth, driving, doing the washing-up and so on. You can literally do anything mindfully! Simply attend to what you are doing, as you are actually doing it. You might want to choose one activity to engage in mindfully per week, and put a post-it note to remind you in the place where the activity gets carried out (on the bathroom mirror, on the washing-up liquid, with the car keys, etc.).

Once you are practised at doing everyday tasks mindfully, apply the technique to some aspect of your diabetes regime, maybe testing your blood glucose, weighing yourself, having your insulin or oral medication. Notice what thoughts, emotions and body experiences occur for you and apply the mindfulness strategies described.

References

de Shazer, Steven (1988). *Clues: Investigating Solutions in Brief Therapy*. W.W. Norton, New York.

Rosenzweig, S., Reibel, D., Greeson, J., Edman, J., Jasser, S., McMearty, K. and Goldstein, B. (2007). Mindfulness-Based Stress Reduction is associated with improved glycemic control in Type 2 diabetes mellitus: A pilot study. *Alternative Therapies*, 13(5), 36–8.

Williams, Mark, Teasdale, John, Segal, Zindel and Kabat-Zinn, Jon (2007). *The Mindful Way through Depression: Freeing Yourself from Chronic Unhappiness*. Guilford Press, New York.

Further Reading

Steven de Shazer (1988). *Clues: Investigating Solutions in Brief Therapy*. W.W. Norton, New York.

P. Gilbert (2009). *The Compassionate Mind*. Constable and Robinson, London.

J. Kabat-Zinn (2004). *Wherever You Go, There You Are: Mindfulness Meditation in Everyday Life*. Piatkus, London.

Bill O'Connell (2005). *Solution-Focused Therapy*. Sage, London.

Mark Williams, John Teasdale, Zindel Segal and Jon Kabat-Zinn (2007). *The Mindful Way through Depression: Freeing Yourself from Chronic Unhappiness*. Guilford Press, New York.

10

Recommended Resources

I hope you have found value in what you have learned in this book. I want to remind you that it is only through practising the principles and skills that you will truly gain the benefits you are looking for. Reading the material alone will only get you so far: it is through doing that you will make true progress. It has been said that the only place you'll find success before work is in the dictionary, and this is just as true for diabetes achievement as it is in any other field of activity.

Listed here is a collection of the resources that I consulted in writing this book: works that I most frequently suggest my own clients make use of, and diabetes organizations which can help you find the answers you are looking for. Please do feel free to contact me at www.PositiveDiabetes.com for further information and advice on any of the topics addressed in this book. I'd be very pleased to hear from you.

Diabetes Charities

Diabetes Research and Wellness Foundation: www.drwf.org.uk/.
Diabetes UK: www.diabetes.org.uk/.
Juvenile Diabetes Research Foundation: www.jdrf.org.uk/.
American Diabetes Association: www.diabetes.org.
Diabetics With Eating Disorders: http://www.dwed.org.uk
Canadian Diabetes Association: http://www.diabetes.ca/
Diabetes Australia: http://www.diabetesaustralia.com.au
European Association for the Study of Diabetes: http://www.easd.org/easd/
International Diabetes Federation: http://www.idf.org/
Hong Kong Juvenile Diabetes Association: http://www.hkjda.org/en/home.html

Diabetes and Wellbeing: Managing the Psychological and Emotional Challenges of Diabetes Types 1 and 2, First Edition. Dr Jen Nash.
© 2013 John Wiley & Sons, Ltd. Published 2013 by John Wiley & Sons, Ltd.

InDependent Diabetes Trust: http://iddt.org
Insulin For Life: http://www.insulinforlifeusa.org
International Society for Paediatric and Adolescent Diabetes: http://www.ispad.org
International Insulin Foundation: http://www.access2insulin.org/
World Diabetes Foundation: http://www.worlddiabetesfoundation.org
Diabetes Ireland: www.diabetes.ie

Education

Dose Adjustment for Normal Eating (DAFNE): www.dafne.uk.com/.
Diabetes Education and Self-Management for Ongoing and Newly Diagnosed (Desmond): www.desmond-project.org.uk/.
Xpert Health: www.xperthealth.org.uk/.
NHS resources: www.nhs.uk/Conditions/Diabetes/Pages/Diabetes.aspx.

Diabetes Supplies

MedicAlert: www.medicalert.org.uk. Supplies identification emblems to alert people to your diabetes.
Desang: www.desang.net/. Produces kitbags.
Joe's Diabetes: www.joes-diabetes.com/.
Diabetes Express: www.diabetesexpress.co.uk/.

Nutrition

Azmina Nutrition: www.azminanutrition.com/.
American Diabetes Association: http://www.diabetes.org/food-and-fitness/food/
Cheyette, C. and Balolia, Y. (2010). *Carbs & Cals: A Visual Guide to Carbohydrate & Calorie Counting for People with Diabetes*. Chello Publishing, London.
NHS Healthy Eating: http://www.nhs.uk/LiveWell/healthy-eating/Pages/Healthyeating.aspx
Nutrition.gov: http://www.nutrition.gov/nutrition-and-health-issues/diabetes
Worral-Thompson, A., Govindji, A. and Suthering, J. (2008). *The Diabetes Weight Loss Diet*. Kyle Cathie. London.

Motivational and Support Resources

Diabetic Friend: http://diabeticfriend.co.uk/.
Joyful Diabetic: www.joyfuldiabetic.com/.
David Mendosa: www.mendosa.com/.
A Sweet Life: www.asweetlife.org
Bitter-Sweet Diabetes: www.bittersweetdiabetes.com
Blue Heel Society: http://blueheelsociety.blogspot.co.uk/

D-Mom: www.d-mom.com
Diabetes Hands Foundation: www.diabeteshandsfoundation.org
Diabetes 24-7: http://www.diabetes24-7.com
Diabetes Mine: http://www.diabetesmine.com/
Diabetes Self-Management: www.diabetesselfmanagement.com
Diabetes Sisters: https://www.diabetessisters.org/
Diabetes Social Media Advocacy Blog: www.diabetessocmed.com
Diabetes Stops Here: www.diabetesstopshere.org
Diabetes Stories: www.diabetesstories.com
Diabetesaliciousness: diabetesaliciousness.blogspot.com
Riva Greenberg's Blog: http://www.huffingtonpost.com/riva-greenberg/
Scott's Diabetes: www.scottsdiabetes.com
Six Until Me: http://www.sixuntilme.com
Tu Diabetes: www.tudiabetes.org
Type 2 Diabetes, A Personal Journal: loraldiabetes.blogspot.com
Texting My Pancreas: www.textingmypancreas.com
World Diabetes Day: http://www.idf.org/worlddiabetesday
Joslin Diabetes Centre: http://www.joslin.org
Successful Diabetes: http://www.successfuldiabetes.com
Positive Diabetes: www.PositiveDiabetes.com
dLife: www.dlife.com/.
Diabetes Daily: www.diabetesdaily.com/.
Diabetes.co.uk: www.diabetes.co.uk/.
Diabetes UK support forum: www.diabetessupport.co.uk/boards/.
BBC Health: www.bbc.co.uk/health/.

Find a Therapist

Positive Diabetes: www.PositiveDiabetes.com.
British Psychological Society, Directory of Chartered Psychologists: www.bps
    .org.uk/bpslegacy/dcp.
RSCPP Find a Therapist Directory: www.rscpp.co.uk/.
British Association for Behavioural and Cognitive Psychotherapy (BABCP): Find a
    Therapist Directory: www.cbtregisteruk.com.
British Association for Counselling and Psychotherapy (BACP): Find a Therapist
    Directory: www.itsgoodtotalk.org.uk/therapists/
Dr Beverly Adler: http://www.askdrbev.com/
London Medical Diabetes: http://www.londonmedical.co.uk/specialties/diabetes
    .aspx

Pharmaceutical Companies Internet Resources

Bayer: www.bayerdiabetes.co.uk.
Lilly Diabetes: www.lillydiabetes.com.

Merck: www.journeyforcontrol.com.
Novo Nordisk: www.novonordisk.co.uk/documents/promotion_page/document
/2007_diabetes_fp_pr.asp.
Sanofi Aventis: www.sanofi.co.uk/l/gb/en/layout.jsp?scat=4E9D46E4-0AE1-4CC9
-8CBF-B8FAB8FB9EF4.

Useful Books

Beverly Adler (2011). *My Sweet Life: Successful Women with Diabetes*. PESI Health
Care, WI.
Beverly Adler (2012). *My Sweet Life: Successful Men with Diabetes*. PESI Health
Care, WI.
Gretchen Becker (2004). *The First Year, Type 2 Diabetes*. Constable and Robinson,
London.
Linda Blair (2008). *Straight Talking*. Piatkus, London.
Gillian Butler and Tony Hope (1995). *Manage Your Mind*. Oxford University Press,
Oxford.
Dennis Greenberger and Christine Padesky (1995). *Mind Over Mood*. Guilford
Press, New York.
William Polonsky (1999). *Diabetes Burnout*. American Diabetes Association,
Alexandria, VA.
Jill Rogers and Rosemary Walker (2010). *Diabetes: A Practical Guide to Managing
Your Health*. Dorling Kindersley, London.
Rubin, Alan and Jarvis, Sarah (2007). *Diabetes for Dummies*. Wiley and Sons,
Chichester.
Schmidt, U. and Treasure, J. (2007). *Getting Better Bit(e) by Bit(e): A Survival Kit
for Sufferers of Bulimia Nervosa and Binge Eating Disorder*. Routledge, Hove.
Stockwell Mercer, Amy (2012). *The Smart Woman's Guide to Diabetes*. Demos
Health, New York.
Vieira, G. (2012). *Emotional Eating with Diabetes: Your Guide to Creating a Positive
Relationship with Food*. Champlain College Publishing, Vermont.
Williams, Mark, Teasdale, John, Segal, Zindel and Kabat-Zinn, Jon (2007). *The
Mindful Way through Depression: Freeing Yourself from Chronic Unhappiness*.
Guilford Press, New York.
Wiseman, Richard (2009). *59 Seconds: Think a Little*, Change a Lot. Macmillan,
London.

Index

Diabetes and Wellbeing: Managing the Psychological and Emotional Challenges of Diabetes Types 1 and 2,
First Edition. Dr Jen Nash.
© 2013 John Wiley & Sons, Ltd. Published 2013 by John Wiley & Sons, Ltd.